THE CAPACITY FOR EMOTIONAL GROWTH

THE CAPACITY FOR EMOTIONAL GROWTH

ELIZABETH R. ZETZEL
M.D., F.R.C.P.

NEW YORK
INTERNATIONAL UNIVERSITIES PRESS, INC.

Library of Congress Catalog Card Number: 71-126355

Printed in Great Britain

CONTENTS

PREFACE

There have been and will continue to be many questions pertaining to the relative importance of internal and external factors in determining individual growth and development. Recent research has highlighted the importance of external stimuli and complex relationships, both gratifying and frustrating, in eliciting positive adaptive efforts towards mastery of internal and external reality. Childhood development, as will be amplified in later chapters, culminates in the recognition that the internal wishes expressed in oedipal fantasies are incompatible with the real affection for both parents already integrated in one-to-one relationships. Not only fear and hate, but also love and trust are prerequisite to mature resolution of this important conflict.

Related considerations may be raised in respect of the emergence and later development of specific areas of interest in professional careers. An apparent conflict of interests was, for example, a major determinant of my initial motivation towards integration of psychoanalytic knowledge within the profession of clinical psychiatry. This conflict was highlighted by the fact that my analytic training was substantially completed before I graduated from medical school. I thus approached psychiatry with the underlying assumption that psychoanalytic knowledge was adequate preparation for the evaluation of patients covering the whole range of clinical psychiatry. This assumption proved, however, to be one which needed considerable modification during the course of my training in psychiatry at the Maudsley Hospital.

This training was largely acquired during the year preceding the outbreak of World War II. I was thus qualified to serve as a psychiatrist in the Emergency Medical Service and the Armed Forces during the six years which followed. On the one hand this represented a considerable interruption of my analytic career. On the other it reinforced my interest in applying psychoanalytic knowledge to the evaluation and treatment of many hundreds of neurotic soldiers. My experiences during these years confirmed my conviction regarding the value of psychoanalytic theory as the basis for the understanding of many psychiatric problems. It also made me aware of significant differences between patients who clearly belonged to the group of transference neurotics and those whose character structure or symptomatology suggested deeper underlying problems.

For these reasons I continued after the end of World War II to apply analytic knowledge at the reconstituted Institute of Psychiatry at the Maudsley Hospital. At the same time I resumed psychoanalytic practice and was appointed Assistant Director of the London Clinic of Psychoanalysis. Before my return to America in 1949 I had given several courses at the London Institute of Psychoanalysis.

I am deeply appreciative of the fact that this volume is appearing under the joint auspices of the International Psycho-Analytical Library and the International Universities Press. Although two-thirds of my professional life has been spent in the United States, my roots will always remain in London where I received both my analytic and my psychiatric training. I should therefore acknowledge my life indebtedness to the late Ernest Jones who introduced me to psychoanalysis, and to the late Eric Guttman who first stimulated my broader interest in clinical psychiatry. I am deeply appreciative of the help I have had from Dr. Donald Winnicott. My first awareness of the importance of early object relations was attributable to my opportunity to work in his Clinic at Paddington Green Hospital. I am also indebted to him for his encouragement in the publication of this volume.

I would also like to express my appreciation to Mr. Masud Khan whose help has been invaluable and to Mr. Joseph Sandler, Editor of the *International Journal of Psycho-Analysis*. I am particularly grateful to him for recommending Mr. Albert Dickson as an editorial assistant. Mr. Dickson's help has been invaluable during the final editing of the manuscript. I am also indebted to him for preparing the Index. Finally, I should like to express my appreciation to my husband, Dr. Louis Zetzel, for his help and encouragement in every aspect of my professional career.

SECTION I

Psychoanalysis and Psychiatry

I

INTRODUCTION

During the years of Freud's pioneer work his approach to psychotic illness represented in essence an attempt to apply the discoveries made in clinical psychoanalysis and dream interpretation to the manifest symptomatology of psychotic patients. His most important contribution in this area, as is well known, did not derive from direct contact with sick patients. He examined rather the journal of a psychotic patient in much the same way that he approached mythology and literature. His concept of narcissism and his approach to mourning and melancholia, although based on certain clinical observations, did not derive from the psychoanalytic treatment of patients suffering from psychotic disorders.

During the early years of the psychoanalytic movement it was Abraham who made the most serious efforts to approach a wide spectrum of mental illness from the point of view of psychoanalysis. His contributions to this subject remain of decisive importance. His attempt, in particular, to correlate different levels of libidinal development with characteristic types of object relationship dominated psychoanalytic efforts to formulate a classification of mental illness for many years. Such an orientation determined the approach to psychosis during my own psychoanalytic training. At that time, moreover, I gained the impression that psychoanalytic theory provided an adequate tool for the diagnosis and evaluation of all psychiatric patients. The then current curriculum in psychiatry for medical students was limited to ten formal demonstrations in a typical state hospital. Apart, therefore, from my own supervised analytic cases, somewhat enriched by presentations at clinical conferences, I had had no contact with psychiatric patients before I commenced my psychiatric training in 1938. It may thus readily be understood that this very one-sided education inevitably led me into serious errors in my initial evaluation of patients in the wards of the Maudsley Hospital.

That I soon recognized this state of affairs is indicated by my recollection after more than twenty-five years of the first patients assigned to me. One of them epitomizes a misuse of psychoanalysis which, even today, leads to serious errors of judgement relevant to the criteria for recommending psychoanalysis and related methods of psychotherapy.

This patient was a young girl admitted in a state of severe turmoil. Always demanding both gratification and her own way, she had recently been involved in an intense quarrel with her parents about a boy-friend. As increasing realistic incompatibilities confronted her, she became confused, resentful and angry, finally accusing her parents of plotting against her. These symptoms had led to a presumptive diagnosis of acute schizophrenia on admission. A few days later, however, when I first saw her, her presenting symptoms had substantially disappeared. She was thus able to give a clear and coherent account of her recent history, with no indication of psychotic ideation. Her major conflicts appeared, moreover, to be almost exclusively at the oedipal level. I therefore discounted her recent decompensation as transient and exaggerated, and reached the conclusion that she was basically neurotic. Since her symptomatology bore evidence to fixation at the oedipal level, she fell within the psychoanalytic classification of hysteria. This diagnosis implied a treatment of choice—namely, psychoanalysis.

Though her rapid remission raised some questions, the initial diagnosis determined her therapy—insulin shock treatment. During the weeks that followed she expanded physically from a rather attractive young woman into a round and flabby butterball. No parallel growth could be discerned in her mental or emotional status. It is probable that this patient was neither an acute schizophrenic nor a straightforward neurotic. Traditional psychoanalysis, like insulin treatment, would not have served her therapeutic needs. It may be noted that physical, like psychological, methods of treatment have been subject to substantial misuse, while their areas of therapeutic efficacy remain subject to investigation.

This experience first alerted me to possible limitations of manifest instinctual content as the primary basis for diagnostic classification. I could not, however, evaluate modes of feeling, thought and perception within the framework of psychoanalytic theory as I then understood it. During the year preceding the outbreak of World War II, I continued to analyse my remaining two control patients. My major efforts were, however, directed towards attaining experience and skill as a clinical psychiatrist. I postponed for the time being any attempt to make sweeping applications of analytic theory to my understanding of the clinical manifestations of different types of mental illness.

During World War II, working first at a Neurosis Centre and later in the R.A.M.C., I was able to confirm my earlier impression that the content or meaning of symptoms in terms of instinctual levels was not sufficient to account for the degree of disability, the natural course of illness or, finally, the response to psychotherapy. My first analytic paper, written in 1943, described the symptomatology and response to treatment of three neurotic soldiers. None of the three was seriously disturbed. All of them were men with a good previous record of achievement, both personal and professional. None of them had experienced the type of separation anxiety described by Fairbairn in a contemporaneous paper. All of them had made a good adjustment to army life up to the time of the specific anxiety-provoking experience. The first, who was the most disturbed, recovered the most rapidly. The second remained mildly depressed. The third, though minimally incapacitated at an objective level, had suffered a relatively irreversible personality change after a traumatic battle experience.

These three cases (referred to in a number of chapters in this volume) serve as a model or blueprint for the areas of my major interest as a psychiatrist and a psychoanalyst. The first patient may, for example, serve as an illustration of a good male hysteric. He was, in brief, a patient who would have profited from traditional psychoanalysis. His history, his symptomatology, his dreams and his self-description bore clear evidence to the fact that, unlike the patient described above, he had indeed attained, but incompletely mastered, a genuine triangular oedipal situation. His phobic symptoms and his manifest anxiety bore evidence to his capacity to recognize and tolerate anxiety. Although at that time the term 'therapeutic alliance' had not entered my vocabulary, it is clear retrospectively that this patient's improvement was primarily attributable to the therapeutic relationship. In the brief period of time available in a War Neurosis Centre, it would not have been possible fully to resolve the transference neurosis which was ready to emerge.

The second patient may also retrospectively be considered as a good example of neurotic (or reactive) depression which illustrates many of the points discussed by Edward Bibring in his important paper, 'The Mechanism of Depression' (1953). Subsequent to his battle experience this patient was confronted by the fact that he was not as good as he had previously believed. His self-esteem was thus impaired; in addition, there was much to indicate that aggression, previously available to the ego for defensive purposes (a reaction formation), had shifted its site of action from ego to superego. The kind of self-reproach and self-depreciation he showed represents a classical example of neurotic depression. The relative chronicity of his condition suggests that his previous adaptation had not been based on genuine mastery of recognized and tolerated depression. It had rather depended on the type of pseudo-mastery described in Chapter 6.

The third case, finally, belonged to the group of wartime neurotics who brought to my attention the prophylactic value against traumatic neurosis of previously acknowledged manifest anxiety. The contrast, in briefest terms, between patients resembling the first and third stimulated my interest in anxiety as a concomitant of the capacity for emotional growth. It should be noted in this context that these specific cases were selected to illustrate typical conditions. By 1943, when my first paper was written, well over one hundred neurotic soldiers had been examined and treated in a War Neurosis Centre. Between that time and the end of the war many more were seen. The clinical material which later resulted in the theoretical paper 'Anxiety and the Capacity to Bear It' (see Chapter 3) was based, as a result, on a very large sample of both male and female neurotic soldiers. This paper was the last I presented in London before returning to my native country in 1949.

At the time I arrived in Boston many attempts had been made to apply techniques closely related to that of traditional psychoanalysis in the treatment of a wide range of psychiatric conditions. During the wave of enthusiasm for psychoanalysis which followed World War II in America, such attempts dominated many psychiatric hospitals. The approach of many inexperienced residents to diagnostic evaluation thus strongly reminded me of my own premature efforts in 1938. The pendulum had swung too far. Premature attempts to achieve integration between psychoanalysis and psychiatry threatened the integrity of both disciplines. I thus found myself playing the part of the devil's advocate. My emphasis on the need for careful formal evaluation often sounded more like Sir Aubrey Lewis at the Maudsley than the deep and exciting psychoanalytic reconstructions which had been hopefully anticipated. In extreme forms, and particularly among those who had had no psychoanalytic training or experience, I met once more the naive conviction that psychiatry and psychoanalysis were not to be distinguished. Criticism of a psychiatry based on blind Freudian faith is not always justified. Such uncritical belief in the total applicability of psychoanalysis is only equalled by its opposite—total rejection. Each position denies the need to undertake the long and difficult tasks involved in the search for areas of genuine communication.

This difficulty may be clarified by the premise that psychiatry inevitably implies a number of different approaches. Some of the implications of this fact were decisively summarized by Lord Brain: 'Recognition that there are different kinds of language in psychiatry will prevent us from making the mistake of believing that the scientific method of verification, however valuable in its own sphere, is universally applicable. Nor', he goes on to say, 'does a system of psychopathological theory necessarily stand or fall by the success or failure of its therapeutic applications' (1963).

Freud's major emphasis at all times was on understanding, irrespective of therapeutic results. He was aware from the outset of the dangers which might follow the search for rapid methods of cure. From a very early period, moreover, he made a relatively sharp distinction between psychosis and neurosis in respect of the capacity to respond to traditional psychoanalytic treatment. Many contemporary psychoanalysts would agree that psychotic patients do not respond to the technique of traditional psychoanalysis. Whatever their theoretical orientation, however, they would maintain that psychoanalytic knowledge has added immeasurably, both to our understanding and to our therapeutic effectiveness in the treatment of patients suffering from serious psychological disorders. This subject will be discussed in more detail in the concluding chapter of this section.

It must be emphasized that Freud's lack of therapeutic

optimism regarding the analytic treatment of psychotic disorders did not diminish his interest in understanding every type of mental illness. At least implicitly he was in full agreement with Lord Brain's 1963 statement. Freud's approach to psychosis was, however, on the whole microscopic rather than macroscopic. His major interest was in examining the instinctual or fantasy meaning of manifest symptomatology in the widest variety of clinical conditions. The continued general validity of some of his observations bears evidence to the fruitfulness of this method of approach. It may nevertheless be suggested that, however valuable this exploration proved to be during the years of pioneer discoveries, it may be subject to the law of diminishing returns over the passage of time. As suggested in relation to my first case illustration, the fact that a patient presents symptoms or fantasies indicative of an unresolved oedipal conflict is not sufficient to justify a diagnosis of an analysable hysterical neurosis (see Chapter 14). In summary, very similar content may be expressed by potentially healthy neurotics at one extreme, and by patients suffering from a schizophrenic disorder at the other.

The approach to psychoanalytic psychiatry implicit in the first section of this volume is macroscopic rather than microscopic. It is based, first, on a consideration of the role of affect tolerance and mastery in determining the predisposition to certain types of psychological disorder. It is based, second, on my increasing conviction of the importance of making both a conceptual and a clinical distinction between instinctual regression limited to neurotic symptom formation or controlled affective distress, and the more serious regression which leads to impairment of basic ego functions. Such regression is not necessarily ominous when it occurs in the setting of developmental crisis or serious stress. It may indeed prove to be transient and reversible with minimal therapeutic intervention. Such regression, which may have progressive implications, must therefore be distinguished from the more insidious regression which characterizes certain forms of psychotic illness.

Whatever its form, regression must in addition be differentiated from developmental failure. Such failures may be relative and partial, as indicated in the chapters on anxiety and depression. It may, however, be more serious and pervasive. Self-object differentiation may be limited or vulnerable. No secure one-to-one relationship may ever have been achieved. There is much to indicate that many individuals, particularly those coming from very limited or deprived emotional backgrounds, may never have experienced a genuine triangular conflict. Such developmental failures may be understood within the framework of psychoanalysis as a comprehensive developmental psychology. They highlight, however, the implications of Lord Brain's statement. Traditional psychoanalysis is the treatment of choice for potentially mature adult patients whose developmental failures are mainly confined to the area of mastery of genuine internal conflict. It is readily to be understood that attempts have been made, and will continue to be made, to use this therapeutic method as the only one which holds out any hope for more severe neurotic disabilities and certain character disorders. Such attempts, however, should not be made with too much therapeutic optimism. They can only succeed if the patient proves to be capable of achieving and maintaining a stable one-to-one relationship in the therapeutic situation.

Serious questions must, however, be raised as to the use of a therapeutic method which fosters regression in the treatment of patients who are clearly handicapped by serious developmental failure. Patients who cannot tolerate anxiety or depression will seldom prove capable of working through a transference neurosis. Many such patients cannot terminate any form of therapy successfully. In approaching the relationship between psychiatry and psychoanalysis, it is essential to make a clear distinction between psychoanalytic understanding which may be utilized in the evaluation of every psychiatric patient and the selection of those patients who can best profit by psychoanalytic treatment and related insight therapy. The development, finally, of methods of therapy other than traditional psychoanalysis based on sound analytic understanding of different clinical conditions remains an area which has not as yet been fully explored. Some of the major considerations integral to this difficult and challenging task will be introduced in the concluding chapter of this section.

2

WAR NEUROSIS: A CLINICAL CONTRIBUTION[1]

(1943)

Most of the analytical material published during and after World War I on the subject of war neurosis dealt with relatively gross disturbances. The attention of the authors at that time was rightly directed towards demonstrating the psychogenic, as opposed to the physiogenic, nature of 'shell shock'. Concentration on demonstrating the psychogenic character in general, however, was unfavourable to the more refined psychological investigation of the individual case. Usually the purpose of the symptoms—namely, to avoid further fighting—was so obvious and so near the surface as barely to merit the description 'unconscious'.

In World War II the clinical material seen by psychiatrists was fundamentally different; crude hysterical reactions were rarer, and anxiety state and depression were the most common clinical diagnoses. It may be because of a lingering memory from the first war that many psychiatrists sought a common aetiological basis for all neuroses in the subsequent war. 'Flight into illness', formerly considered the common cause of all neuroses, may therefore soon be replaced by 'separation anxiety'. Instead of fear of the battlefield, some speak of 'lack of morale and social conscience', and the moralistic attitude goes so far that a member of the British Psycho-Analytical Society has stated: 'Perhaps it is small wonder that after acquiring some disillusioning experience of neurotic service men *en masse* I was driven to remark, "What these people really need is not a psychotherapist but an evangelist"' (Fairbairn, 1943, p. 287).

The operation of general (group) factors such as lack of morale in the origin of war neuroses cannot be denied; indeed my experience at a Neurosis Centre impressed me with the importance of constitutional and environmental factors in bringing about

[1] Paper read before the British Psycho-Analytical Society on 3 March 1943 and first published in the *Int. J. Psycho-Anal.* (1943), **24**.

neurotic reactions of a purely escapist type at a conscious or preconscious level. However, broad statements about such cases contribute little to our knowledge of the unconscious, and dogmatic statements which suggest that we have little to learn from war neuroses have been based on premature generalization.

Unconscious conflicts are equally important for all individuals, well or ill, and the borderline between health and illness is not a sharp one; but there are great individual differences in the capacity to bear instinctual tension and anxiety. Among military cases there are a great many chronic neurotics who have never been able to stand up to tension and frustration. Analytic investigation of such cases, interesting as it would be at the deepest levels, would yield little information concerning the specific psychogenesis of the current war neurosis. Most men who break down shortly after joining the army belong to this category, and there is no point in labelling them war neurotics at all. Many other cases of apparently acute breakdown also reveal, on psychiatric investigation, that the current neurosis is only a new expression of a lifelong inadequacy. Still, frequent as such observations may be, they do not cover the whole range of clinical material. There is, in particular, a small but by no means negligible group of men with *no* previous history of personality maladjustment or inadequacy, who nevertheless have broken down after actual battle experience.

The study of such cases has some bearing on another problem. It is not many years since Freud commented on the remarkable fact that we are even yet not in a position to answer the apparently simple question of why one person develops a neurosis and another not. Analytic practice in peace time is mostly concerned with chronic cases or with patients so severely disturbed that neurotic illness appears inevitable in retrospect. It is probably for this reason that Edward Glover said, in concluding his notes on the psychological effects of war conditions on the civilian population: 'The most fruitful line of investigation . . . will probably lie in the full analysis of minor, delayed and vestigial types' (1942, p. 37).

The observations to be discussed in this chapter follow on this line of thought. They comprise three cases of relatively mild neurosis in previously healthy men. This type of case is easily forgotten by the statistically orientated psychiatrist on account of its numerical insignificance; but it offers to the psychoanalyst, interested in the individual case, material of some importance in regard to general theory.

Conditions of work in a busy Neurosis Centre make full analysis, even in selected cases, impossible, but the wealth of clinical material enables the analytically trained psychiatrist to select outstanding cases for more detailed, though still limited investigation, and to view findings in the individual case against the background of the general psychogenesis and psychopathology in large numbers of others.

In this chapter, therefore, I propose to illustrate some theoretical questions by means of material drawn from three cases of relatively mild neurosis in previously well-adjusted personalities. The fact that all these men were in the army explains their admission to hospital—none of them was sufficiently ill to have sought hospital treatment under the conditions of civilian life, and it was only because their symptoms prevented them from fulfilling combatant duties that they had been referred to psychiatrists. None of these men had previously regarded himself as nervous and they had all led lives in which there was little or no objective evidence of serious mental conflict. They were all happily married; they all had a steady work record; they had all shown ambition, social conscience and a good capacity for sublimation. They had all made a good adjustment to army life and they had all broken down after specific war experiences—the first after air-raid experiences in England, the other two following evacuation from Dunkirk. They had also all continued on full duty for at least a year after their experiences prior to admission to hospital.

In spite of the superficial similarities enumerated, it will be seen that these three cases present considerable variation in psychogenesis and psychopathology. Each of these, that is to say, fell ill for a different reason—although, in each case, war experiences had precipitated a neurotic illness which otherwise might not have appeared. Does the way in which these experiences were utilized throw any light on the origin of neurotic illness?

Among other questions raised by these cases are the following:

(1) Is there any justification for recent statements that war neurosis is due to 'separation anxiety' in unduly dependent men?

(2) Does the diagnosis 'anxiety state', which had been given to all these men, imply a similar psychopathology?

(3) Does the aggressive instinct play a specific aetiological role in the psychogenesis of certain war neuroses?

(4) What is the psychopathology of the depression so frequently observed in cases of war neurosis?

Needless to say, I do not expect to give definite answers to all these questions in this chapter. I mention them as problems to keep in mind in considering the clinical material.

Case 1. Private A., aged twenty-six, was admitted to hospital in March 1942, complaining of nervousness and insomnia of over a year's duration, dating from experiences in air-raids a year before.

A. was the third child of an unsuccessful professional jockey and had earned his own living from a very early age. He had always been cheerful, active and self-reliant and had not regarded himself as at all nervous, although he had been enuretic to the age of fourteen, had walked in his sleep and bitten his nails. He was very small, and in his childhood had been teased a good deal because of an unusually large head.

Ambitious, energetic, and somewhat aggressive, he had progressed rapidly in his chosen trade—and by the time he was twenty-four had been earning between seven and ten pounds a week as the manager of a successful restaurant. . . . His sexual activities had also proved satisfactory, though somewhat lacking in tenderness; he had had successful affairs and had then made a happy marriage at the age of twenty-two. He had one child aged two.

He was called up in May 1940, and settled down well to army life. His catering knowledge was soon recognized by his officers and he was congenially employed in the officers' mess, with excellent chances of promotion.

During the winter of 1940–41 he was posted in a town which had some extremely heavy air-raids, and volunteered for work on a rescue squad. He was knocked over by blast several times, saw many horrible sights, and frequently helped in the removal of maimed and dismembered bodies. He became somewhat anxious towards the end of the blitz but did not report sick. His unit moved to another part of the country, where he remained on full duty. Some time about June, however, he noticed that he was still very tense and restless. He was also sleeping badly and had numerous disturbing nightmares. He reported sick and was given a short period of leave without improvement. He was then referred to a psychiatrist, who recommended that he should remain on duty in a lower medical grade. He showed no improvement, however, and finally, in March 1942, he was admitted to hospital.

On admission to hospital this man was by far the most incapacitated by his symptoms of the three cases under discussion. He was noticeably tense, anxious and worried about himself. The most striking thing about him was his desire to discuss his difficulties. He said that he had been longing for an opportunity to talk about his problems and to understand them. He knew his illness was psychological in origin and could not understand why he had become ill. To use his own words: 'I could not understand why, after a blitz in which I did a little rescue work, this should affect me in any way, for always since my childhood I had developed a hard, aggressive nature.'

He described dreams which made it clear that his illness had a specific psychogenesis. All his dreams were concerned—not with bombs, bombed places or bombed people—but with aeroplanes and people falling out of them. In particular he described a recent recurrent dream in which he saw a woman in a white dress fall out of a plane and 'float down to earth' without a parachute. He heard his own voice say 'This one's going' and then found the woman lying with her legs folded under her, behind a nearby hedge.

Although I was unable to analyse this dream fully, the patient's associations to it, during my first interview with him, threw a good deal of light on the psychopathology of his neurosis.

The most important associations to the dreams were as follows:

(1) He had been puzzled by the fact that his dreams concerned aeroplanes rather than bombs, but said that he had always been extremely interested in feats of daring in the air, and had been particularly interested in a certain stunt parachute jumper who had finally been killed on an occasion when his parachute had failed to open.

(2) This led him to comment on the fact that he had always been fascinated and frightened by heights. On one occasion he had climbed to the top of a tower to stand on the very spot

where a man had recently made a successful suicidal jump.

(3) The position in which he had found the woman—with legs folded—brought two memories. First, of an occasion in his boyhood when he had seen a girl lose control of her bicycle on a steep hill and fall off in a similar position with severe disfiguring injuries. He had helped her to call an ambulance but had not dared make further enquiries although he had been very much interested. Second, he recalled that his father had had numerous falls—particularly in steeplechases—and that he had seen him fall during a race in his early childhood.

(4) While recounting these memories, he said something very important had come into his mind, namely, that his severe anxiety symptoms dated—not from the general experiences during the air-raids, which had not disturbed him more than his companions—but from a single incident which had upset him considerably. He had been asked to help remove the bodies of several Dutch airmen who had recently been killed in a crash. He touched the body of one of them and found that it was still warm. This filled him—to use his own words—with 'unspeakable horror'—and it was from this incident that his severe anxiety symptoms dated.

In the very short treatment which followed, the patient continued to show richness of associations and a desire to understand—combined with unusual psychological insight. I will summarize the points of chief importance which emerged and then discuss the case as a whole.

I learned that at the time of these air-raids he had become very friendly with an older married couple who lived in the town. He had at first been equally friendly with husband and wife, but had gradually found himself on more affectionate terms with the woman, who apparently took a somewhat maternal interest in him. The husband had gone into the army only a short time before the raids began—and, although the patient was sure there was nothing 'wrong' in his friendship with the woman, he began to feel a little doubtful about it. He had broken off this friendship shortly after the onset of his symptoms.

He discussed his sexual life freely, and without much interpretation connected some former aggressive over-confidence with his earlier feelings of inferiority about his size and his head in a way which would have delighted an Adlerian. To quote again from the account he wrote for me about his illness: 'Now for the sexual side. I rather gather that the sexual instinct is one of the most dominant factors in the average human being. I know it can be the means of expressing one's failings and triumphs. Aggressiveness is one way it can be expressed. I would also say it could express the inferiority complex in this way: the sexual organ can be used as an aggressive force, giving an almost brutal tendency, and so bluff the individual into believing he has not got an inferiority complex; or it could, in the case of physical defect, tend to make up for the thing which is lacking in the individual.'

It did not appear that his sexual potency with his wife had been affected in any noticeable degree during the course of his illness. On the other hand, his self-confidence in dealing with other men had been materially impaired and he had lost a great deal of his former interest in his work. He felt himself that he had 'lost' his former aggressiveness—he had also lost a good deal of his interest in the army and the war—and was very apprehensive about future experiences of enemy action. In this connection his fear was specific. He wrote:

> Now on one occasion I had to come into contact with a dead airman. My horror was unspeakable on finding that he was still warm. Yet I had handled many bodies previous to this. When I saw the result of the crash, coupled with the terrible cases I had seen during the blitz, it shattered my aggressiveness. Is this a form of cowardice? My thoughts on seeing all this violence turn to myself and my family. I have one horror and one fear during this war and that is the thought of losing a limb.

The symbolic meaning of this fear is obvious. Its fundamental importance in the precipitation of his neurosis was confirmed in the course of his treatment. The turning point of his illness was reached when in his associations he revived, with considerable emotion, a previously forgotten experience of horror which he described as exactly similar to his feeling on touching the dead airman. This was an occasion in his childhood when he had been helping his father with some ferrets he owned. He had seen that one of the ferrets was suffering from a disease known as 'tail rot', and had been overwhelmed by a feeling of fear and disgust.

During his stay in hospital the patient attended physical

training, which was held on the floor of an indoor swimming pool with the instructor standing on the edge of the basin above the class. During the course of his treatment A. frequently commented on the anxiety this situation caused him. He was constantly torn, he told me, between a desire and a fear that the instructor should fall off the edge. This conflicting attitude had also been shown by his previous interest in people (such as stunt fliers) who took constant risks and by his fascination (as shown by his climbing the tower) in fatal falls. When it is remembered that his father had been a jockey who frequently fell, it does not seem unjustifiable to suggest that his attitude towards heights was related to ambivalent feelings about his father. The desire that he should fall represented a death wish in the classical Oedipus situation.

The psychopathology and psychogenesis of this case raise many interesting problems. It is of course impossible to know the whole story as the treatment was very limited. It seemed to me, however, that the case provided an unusually clear picture of the reappearance in adult life of an infantile neurosis at the height of the Oedipus conflict. At the time of the war experiences, he had been involved in an emotional situation which recalled to his own mind his earlier relationship with his parents. The resolution of his infantile situation had not been complete, in that he had shown anxiety symptoms throughout childhood. He had also been left with a mild phobia about heights, and his fear of castration had been overcompensated by an aggressive faith in infallible sexual potency. It was abundantly clear that his main anxiety was related to castration fear. The contact with the body of the dead airman (whatever deeper meaning it may have had) appeared to have reactivated this specific fear—as shown by his conscious terror of mutilation by losing a limb. At the same time, his former solution (namely, over-confidence and lack of tenderness) no longer appeared to be open to him. It is possible that the knowledge that the airman was actually dead—associated as it was with real experiences which constantly emphasized and reiterated the existence of real external danger and hostility—made his former defence of relative omnipotence and lack of fear in relation to other men untenable. We did not reach any deeper guilt concerning his omnipotent death wishes except by inference.

Although this man was clinically the most ill of the three patients under consideration, he made by far the best recovery. His illness was of particular interest because of the way in which his air-raid experiences had touched upon unresolved conflicts associated with the classical Oedipus situation. . . . Although—or perhaps some of us might say because—he had throughout his life been accustomed to dealing with anxiety associated with his genital demands, his experiences did not fundamentally alter his most important human relationships. He did not, like the other men I shall discuss, lose any capacity for object relationships. He showed little depression. His sexual potency was not affected, and, in spite of continued mild anxiety and slight subjective loss of self-confidence, he remained a fundamentally cheerful, friendly and ambitious little man who went back to the army with the renewed intention of earning promotion.

Case 2. Sergeant B., a regular soldier aged twenty-six, was admitted to hospital in March 1942, complaining of loss of self-confidence and undue fatigability of about eighteen months' duration.

B. was the eldest child and only son of an unhappy marriage. All his earliest affection had been directed towards his father, who after failing in business deserted his wife and children, when B. was eleven years old. B. appears to have been a normal child and could not recall any neurotic traits or difficulties. In spite of his great fondness for his father, he had felt no conscious resentment or grief at his departure and had easily adjusted himself to the new situation.

At the age of fifteen he joined the army against his mother's wish and had served continuously ever since. He began as a band boy and had played in the regimental band up to the outbreak of war. He had received steady promotion and had always been well adjusted to army life—on good terms with superiors and inferiors—and very much identified with the history and record of his regiment, which is famous for its fighting qualities.

He married in September 1939, and his first baby was born in June 1941. His marriage was happy and there had been no sexual difficulties in his relationship with his wife, who had been living near him since his return from Dunkirk.

He went to France soon after the outbreak of war and his unit went into action after the invasion of Belgium. Although a little apprehensive before going into battle, he found that he thoroughly enjoyed the fighting, using both bayonet and rifle with considerable gusto during the retreat to Dunkirk. He waited on the beach for over twenty-four hours, and was subjected to numerous dive-bombing attacks which aroused considerable anxiety. He was finally rescued, almost the only one of his group of friends to return safely to England.

For several months after his return he had typical anxiety dreams about dive-bombing which gradually subsided. He did not report sick, however, and continued to get on well in the army; he was promoted in June 1940 and was employed as Intelligence Sergeant to the complete satisfaction of his officers up to the time of his admission to hospital.

In about October 1940 he began to notice that he felt very tired most of the time. His anxiety dreams had vanished and he was sleeping very well, too well in fact, as he never wanted to get up in the morning and also felt that he needed a sleep after his midday dinner. He also noticed that he felt less self-confident in his dealings with other men; he often felt that he was being criticized and found it difficult to give orders effectively. He felt mildly depressed, lost his appetite, and began to lose weight. Nevertheless, he continued on full duty, and was expecting to go abroad. He hoped that under conditions of active service his symptoms would disappear. In January 1942, however, he had an attack of diarrhoea and passed a little blood and mucus. He was therefore admitted to a general hospital for investigation. His lethargy and undue fatigability were noticed; and after all physical investigations had proved negative he was referred to a psychiatrist who recommended his transfer to a Neurosis Centre.

On admission to hospital he was found to be a tall, thin man, with hollow cheeks and fair curly hair, who was extremely intelligent and co-operative and fully accepted the fact that there was nothing physically wrong with him. He admitted that war had seemed rather senseless to him since his experiences at Dunkirk; on the other hand, he denied that this affected his attitude to the army, since he still regarded himself as a regular soldier who intended to serve his full time and hoped to become a sergeant-major or warrant officer in due course. There was little depressive content in his mental state, although he gave the impression of being mildly depressed and uninterested. He talked in a rather monotonous voice with little expression. He admitted that he had changed a great deal since returning from Dunkirk. He showed no overt anxiety, although he said that he sometimes felt nervous when he heard aeroplanes flying low. He described mild ideas of reference, saying that he had occasionally felt that other men were talking about him or laughing at him. His general attitude, however, was not in any way paranoid.

It was not possible to treat this man by an analytic method. He was seen a number of times, however, and considerable light was thrown on the psychogenesis and psychopathology of his illness. The following were the points of chief importance:

(1) The loss of his father had, of course, had a far more important traumatic effect than was obvious at the time. He had successfully repressed a great deal of anger and hatred—both against his father for going, and also against his mother for her failure to hold him.

(2) Although he did not admit to any overt homosexual relations with his fellow soldiers, he had had several very close friendships. He also talked a good deal about the leader of the regimental band who had taken considerable paternal interest in him during his earlier years of military service.

(3) He felt considerable guilt about the fact that he had actually enjoyed fighting. He had never regarded himself as blood-thirsty or aggressive and had felt apprehensive before going into battle. The fact that he had obtained real gratification during the battle was very disturbing to him.

(4) It also appeared that he had completely forgotten his wife for several days during the retreat to Dunkirk. This seemed inconceivable and alarming to him in retrospect.

(5) He felt both self-reproach and considerable grief concerning the loss of his friends. He felt that he ought not to have come back safely without them. Although on the one hand he felt that his return obliged him to do everything possible for his regiment, on the other hand both his retrospective guilt about his gratification and the loss of his friends had brought about a good deal of conscious dislike of war which he could not overcome.

In opening this chapter, I commented on the fact that most of the psychiatric literature of World War I was concerned with gross escapist reactions in unwilling soldiers. It is therefore interesting to find that so much guilt and self-reproach should have followed actual combat in a professional soldier. There appears little doubt that, during the campaign, profound changes took place in this man's mental economy, resulting in an enormous release of formerly repressed aggressive tendencies. It is interesting to speculate whether this could be considered as an example of aggression in pure form. Ernest Jones writes:

> Nevertheless the nosological status of this instinct is by no means clear. Freud holds that the 'tendency to aggression is an innate, independent, instinctual disposition in man', and if the accent is here laid on the word 'tendency' no analyst could doubt the statement, since nothing could appear in fact unless there were a tendency to it. More difficult is the question whether such a tendency ever expresses itself spontaneously and in a pure form. That is to say, would anyone, child or adult, ever make an attack with the intent to injure and destroy unless the impulse was either associated with an erotic one, as it constantly is in sadism, or was a reaction to some thwarting or privation that he finds unendurable? . . . it is extraordinarily difficult to detect spontaneous activity of the aggressive instinct in isolation, and I do not myself know of any unequivocal example (1936, p. 169).

The fact that the patient felt disturbing guilt about aggression which was so thoroughly justified externally as legitimate fighting during a bitter campaign suggests that its significance was complicated. His self-reproach also suggests that a large sadistic element had been present. Two other facts—namely that there was a good deal to suggest strong emotional ties with his friends and that he completely forgot the existence of his wife during the campaign—suggest that this sadism was of a homosexual nature.

Whatever the deeper unconscious aspects of this neurosis, the superficial conflict was clearly between his loyalty to his regiment and his ambitions as a soldier on the one hand and his reaction of guilt and self-reproach to actual battle on the other. It seems clear also that, although there was no evidence of previous neurotic disability, he was predisposed to a neurotic breakdown in that his choice of the army as a career had been determined by unconscious conflicts and a partially homosexual solution of his Oedipus complex. It must be stressed, in conclusion, that this man was never severely incapacitated by his symptoms, which on the whole expressed the increased difficulty and greater cost of maintaining his adjustment. His subjective feeling of lack of energy and undue fatigability were due to the subsequent loss of free psychic energy.

Case 3. Sapper C., a man of thirty-three, was admitted to hospital in May 1942, complaining of depression and a feeling that there was something inside him which made him want to cry. His symptoms were of two years' duration, dating from the retreat to Dunkirk.

He had had no previous psychological difficulties. He came from a Welsh mining district. He was one of a number of children and there was no family history of a nervous or mental illness. His childhood had been happy and normal. He had done well at school and had always been active in athletic and social activities. Like most Welshmen he was musical and had always taken part in concerts. After leaving school he had worked in a quarry and had been employed with the same firm for thirteen years. He was skilled at his work and had been foreman in charge of a hydraulic engine for several years before the war. He had also taken a keen interest in social and economic questions and had been secretary of the local branch of the Labour Party for several years. He had been happily married for eleven years and had two healthy children. He was a strong, well-built man, and had had no serious physical illnesses.

He joined the Supplementary Reserve (a pool of qualified tradesmen) in the spring of 1939 and was called up for active service at the outbreak of war. He went to France with one of the early contingents of the British Expeditionary Force. During the winter of 1939–40 he thoroughly enjoyed army life. He was on good terms with the other members of his unit, took part in various concert parties, did work of a constructional kind in the British Sector and looked forward, with confident anticipation and no anxiety, to active fighting.

His unit went into Belgium at the beginning of the campaign, and being engineers were chiefly employed in blowing up bridges during the retreat. They were subjected to constant and heavy dive-bombing. Early in the retreat a land-mine exploded very near him. Soon, to his own surprise and horror, he found that he was terrified. His nervousness increased rapidly; at the same time he developed a skin condition of his thighs which made it increasingly difficult for him to walk. He began to tremble, and his pitiable state of terror soon became so obvious that his companions took his rifle away from him. His own written description of his experience is self-explanatory:

> The first bridge to be charged was at La Scarpe, then on to a place 7 kilo from Amiens, when my skin was beginning to get raw. During that time and up to the time of leaving, my life was one hell. . . . Near the bottom of Mont Cassel where I was lying on my stomach with fright from the bombing, one dropped quite near and threw me a short distance which resulted in my finding myself crying. From there on I was carried about, until we had to abandon the lorry about twelve miles from Dunkirk.

After the lorry had been abandoned he was unable to keep up with the others, with the result that he sat alone by the roadside in abject terror for nearly twelve hours before he was rescued and brought back to England.

> After being back a few weeks at Sheffield a telegram came to tell me that my mother was very ill, so I was sent home for two days. I found that my mother had passed away, so I returned back to Sheffield late and was put on a charge.

His skin condition improved rapidly, he was again graded A1, and remained on full duty. For various reasons, however, he had not been fully employed in his own trade since his return to England, and, although he had recently passed an advanced course, he had been employed chiefly on routine duties after its completion.

Ever since his return from France he had felt depressed. Although he felt great sorrow after his mother's death, he did not feel that this in any way explained his depression. At times he found himself crying, without knowing why. He was frightened of air-raids. He occasionally found that he felt better after drinking, and for a short time drank fairly heavily, but then gave it up. He had felt too ashamed of his symptoms to report sick for a considerable time. At the same time he had lost all trust in officers and N.C.O.s since his experience of sitting alone by the roadside, followed by the punishment after his mother's death, which he had felt to be unjust. His relationship with his wife was unchanged, and he was not aware of any diminution of his sexual potency.

On admission to hospital he was very much on the defensive; he was afraid of being regarded as a malingerer and, at first, was reluctant to discuss his experiences. Later he was extremely co-operative. His constant and reiterated complaint was that there was something inside him, causing his depression and making him want to cry. It was not easy, however, to ascertain whether by this 'something' he meant something added or something lost, since he frequently stated that he had lost something at Dunkirk which could never be regained. The only thing which could help, he said, was the opportunity to do really useful work again as a skilled tradesman.

After several interviews I came to the conclusion that the origin of the depression lay at too deep a level to make a limited analytic approach advisable. The patient was chiefly helped by the fact that I supported his desire to do useful work by getting him a suitable posting in his own trade. He also joined in group discussions about general psychological problems with some benefit. In spite of the limited material, however, it seems to me that this case raises many points of theoretical interest.

(1) There can be little doubt that this man's whole history was that of a 'normal' man in every sense of the word. His previous adjustment to both sexes had been satisfactory, he had an excellent work record and had also shown considerable capacity for sublimation. His patriotism and high morale are also indicated by the fact that he had volunteered for the Supplementary Reserve although he was in a reserved occupation. In addition he had made a good adjustment to army life before the campaign.

(2) The nature of the traumatic events merits further comment. The exciting incidents appear to have been cumulative. The first event was the near explosion of the land-mine which lifted him off the ground. This appears to have roused anxiety symptoms of a severe kind at the outset. I have elsewhere attempted to relate the traumatic effect of experiences of this type—that is to say, experiences in which the individual is lifted or blown over by blast without injury—to a previous unconscious conviction of invulnerability. This man's complete lack of apprehension before going into action suggests that some such mechanism may have played a part in his case. He was, that is

to say, psychologically unprepared for his experience of fear. To quote Freud:

> The individual will have made an important advance in his capacity for self-preservation if he can foresee and expect a traumatic situation of this kind which entails helplessness, instead of simply waiting for it to happen. Let us call a situation which contains the determinant for such an expectation a danger-situation (1926, p. 166).

If I understand Freud's meaning correctly, it should be legitimate to explain this man's subsequent reaction of increasing fear and helplessness as a repetition of a 'traumatic' as opposed to a 'danger' situation. In this connection the following quotation is also relevant:

> On the other hand, the external (real) danger must also have managed to become internalized if it is to be significant for the ego. It must have been recognized as related to some situation of helplessness that has been experienced. Man seems not to have been endowed, or to have been endowed to only a very small degree, with an instinctive recognition of the dangers that threaten him from without (1926, p. 168).

The symbolic meaning of the second traumatic event—the removal of his rifle—is obvious. In discussing this incident with the patient, however, it was difficult to be certain how important it had been, because of his complete disintegration by the time it happened.

His feeling that he had been deserted by the roadside was, in his own opinion, by far the worst experience of all. To it he ascribed his loss of trust in humanity, his sense of having lost something and his feeling that he could never be the same man again. The subsequent death of his mother, followed by punishment for returning late, had apparently deepened, confirmed and underlined his sense of loss.

What was the nature of this trauma, following as it did an acute anxiety state, complete psychic helplessness and a symbolic castration, and occurring in a setting of continued helplessness, both psychological and physical—it will be remembered that the condition of his legs made it difficult for him to walk—and in the presence of continued and increasing external danger? Could it be regarded as an approximation to that most dreaded infantile situation in which the individual feels himself abandoned by all love objects and in danger of annihilation?

(3) It is interesting to contrast this man's reaction with that of Sergeant B. who had enjoyed the same battle. Whereas in Sergeant B. repressed aggression had been liberated, in Sapper C. the appearance of aggression in any form was conspicuous by its complete absence. It is interesting to speculate concerning the cause of this failure. How was it related to the unconscious determinants of his psychological unpreparedness for the experience of fear? And to what extent was the danger situation internalized during the critical period? It is obviously impossible to answer these questions without further detailed analytic investigation at a deep level.

(4) In this connection it is also important to remember that C.'s presenting symptom two years later was persistent depression. Most analysts would agree that the typical self-depreciation of melancholia is related to aggression directed towards the ego. This man, however, was not melancholic. He ate and slept well. He was friendly and sociable in the ward and always ready to sing at hospital concerts. He had no difficulty in concentration, and during his stay in hospital attended an engineering course where he worked well and with intelligent interest. Nevertheless he was definitely and persistently depressed; although friendly, he showed little spontaneous pleasure. He was often found lying on his bed on pass days. Occasionally he cried. He continued to complain of something inside him which made him miserable and unhappy.

The psychopathology of this case is not, therefore, readily comparable with that of the type of case referred to by Freud (1917) and Karl Abraham (1911) in their papers on melancholia. There was not a complete withdrawal of libido, nor was there the typical self-depreciation of psychotic depression.

The depression, nevertheless, was associated with definite object loss, as was shown by his altered feeling towards his fellow soldiers. The mental state, however, appeared nearer to that of the mourner than to that of true melancholia. Melanie Klein uses another term, which, I think, well describes this man's affective state:

The second set of feelings which go to make up the depressive position I formerly described without suggesting a term for them. I now propose to use for these feelings of sorrow and concern for the loved objects, the fears of losing them and the longing to regain them, a simple word derived from everyday language—namely the 'pining' for the loved object (1940, p. 316).

It is difficult to account for this man's illness except in the terms of very early danger situations. It will be remembered that I was unable to obtain any suggestive evidence concerning previous experiences involving psychological conflict. In addition, his complete helplessness—both psychological and physical—during the campaign is highly suggestive. I have no wish to be dogmatic and I realize that the clinical material available in this case is very limited. My own idea of the psychogenesis of this illness, however, is based on the assumption that the traumatic experiences had reactivated the earliest anxiety situations with subsequent helplessness. This helplessness was also related to internalization of the danger situation. The subsequent depression could thus correspond with Melanie Klein's description of the infantile depressive position: 'In short—persecution (by 'bad' objects) and the characteristic defences against it, on the one hand, and pining for the loved ('good') object on the other, constitute the depressive position' (1940, p. 316). The patient's desire for constructive work could also be explained in terms of ideas of reparation and an attempt to re-create a shattered inner world.

Although clinically the least ill, in that he had no incapacitating symptoms, this man was the most profoundly disturbed of the three cases I have presented. His illness interested me particularly as an example of how vulnerable an apparently completely normal man may be when external experiences combine to arouse his most deeply buried primitive fears.

In this chapter I have selected three cases of relatively mild neurosis appearing in men of previously good mental health following battle experiences. Similar cases, although relatively infrequent, are by no means rare: of two hundred soldiers admitted to my ward during the first eight months of last year nearly 10 per cent were of this type.

It is obvious that in spite of the superficial similarity which made it legitimate to include them in the same clinical group the three patients present very different problems in psychopathology. The first presented symptoms of anxiety associated with phobias of a predominantly genital nature brought about by a reactivation of his oedipal conflict; the second had reacted with guilt and anxiety after the release of formerly repressed aggressive and sadistic impulses; the third presented depressive symptoms following experiences which appear to have approximated to a repetition of some primal traumatic situation.

It is worth noting, also, that these cases illustrate the fact that the presence of anxiety symptoms, both in childhood and in adult life, is often of good prognostic significance. The first man had shown anxiety and a good capacity for its toleration; the second had shown slight anxious anticipation before going into battle; the third could remember no anxiety at all. The first man made a complete recovery from his acute symptoms, although he was left with his fear of heights; the second improved considerably, although he did not regain his former unquestioning adjustment to a male community; the third showed little real change. Although clinically the least ill of the three, this man had undergone the most profound subjective change.

I should like to offer my own very tentative answers to the questions I asked in my introduction:

Is there any justification for recent publications which imply that all war neurosis is due to 'separation anxiety' in unduly dependent men?—It is hardly necessary to repeat that my answer to this question is emphatically in the negative. While there is every reason for indicating that such factors play a part in the appearance of symptoms in men who have shown their inferior capacity to stand average adverse conditions prior to military service, it is ludicrous to suppose that every man who reports sick with symptoms of anxiety or depression after battle experiences is a weakling trying to evade his duty and return home. Such statements, if carried to their logical conclusion, would imply that neurotic illness, following experiences which have been traumatic for the individual, is chiefly due to constitutional inferiorities and hardly worth treating except by moral exhortations and social measures.

(2) Does the diagnosis 'anxiety state', which had been given to

all these men, imply a similar psychopathology?—This is the most common diagnosis given to the neurotics of World War II. Many non-analytic psychiatrists appear to believe that the appearance of anxiety is simply an indication that the individual is a constitutionally anxious man, and that the diagnosis is self-explanatory. No psychoanalyst would maintain such a view, and these cases, it seems to me, clearly indicate that anxiety may be a presenting symptom in neuroses of very different psychological structure.

(3) Does the aggressive instinct play a specific aetiological part in the psychogenesis of certain war neuroses?—The second patient illustrates the problem I have in mind. I have seen other similar cases. It would be surprising if the inevitable release of aggressive impulses in active warfare failed to produce more or less pathological reactions of anxiety and guilt. The point of chief interest in the case quoted was that this reaction should have appeared in a regular soldier, whose profession, after all, was fighting.

(4) What is the psychopathology of the depression so frequently observed in cases of war neurosis?—What relation has this question to the preceding one? The second patient, Sergeant B., who felt guilty about his aggressive gratification, was only very mildly depressed. The third man, Sapper C., who was a typical example of the type of depression I have in mind, had conspicuously failed to show any aggression at all. What part did this failure play in his subsequent depression? It is at least arguable, in view of his conscious realization that something had gone wrong 'inside him', that the situation of external danger had been internalized with subsequent retreat to a depressive position. Why this should have happened it is impossible to say. Many cases of depression following war experiences may be due to a similar internalization of aggressive impulses which could not—either for external or internal reasons—be allowed to express themselves in action.

Lastly, what light do these cases throw on the reason why one person develops a neurosis and another not?—Each of these men fell ill, and, I think, had previously remained well, for different reasons. The first had remained well because of his capacity to bear a considerable amount of anxiety concerned with unresolved elements of his oedipal situation. A specific traumatic experience increased his anxiety until it became pathological, but with little qualitative change in his personality structure or in his capacity for object relationships. The second man had remained well because his chosen career allowed him considerable gratification of his unconscious homosexual impulses. He broke down when battle experiences revealed to him the sadism and aggression underlying his previous adjustment. It is important to note, however, that in spite of considerable subjective change, there was little objective evidence of real neurotic illness and a good deal to indicate that his symptoms were chiefly indicative of the greater cost of maintaining his equilibrium. It is a matter for definition whether such a condition should be diagnosed as a real illness or not. The third case is the most difficult, and I very much regret the impossibility of undertaking full analysis which would, I feel sure, have given invaluable material. The fact that this man, whose previous history offered no clues to potential weak spots, who had no memory of previous anxiety or depression, should have collapsed into such abject helplessness early in the campaign certainly suggests that his normal adjustment had been dependent on a very complete repression of his earliest anxiety situations. To what extent this is true of normal people, it is, of course, impossible to say. From my clinical experience, I am inclined to think that complete so-called normality often has a pathological background.

Although, therefore, I cannot make any general conclusions on the answer to this question, these cases illustrate the fact that normal men may have hidden neurotic potentialities but that external events, no matter how overwhelming, precipitate a neurosis only when they touch on specific unconscious conflicts.

3

ANXIETY AND THE CAPACITY TO BEAR IT[1]

(1949)

There have been few attempts to correlate the premises on which much modern work on anxiety has been based with earlier theoretical formulations regarding its psychopathology. Accordingly, the first aim in this chapter is to review briefly the history and development of analytic thought regarding the nature of anxiety in order to state as clearly as possible those aspects of theory which, although still incomplete, appear to be relatively non-controversial, in so far as they are compatible with considerable differences of opinion in respect of other basic concepts. I also wish to define, particularly with regard to the nature and origin of internal danger situations, other important theoretical concepts which appear far more controversial and about which differences of opinion give rise to unavoidable theoretical controversy.

Owing to the fact that my own interest in this subject was originally stimulated by my opportunity during the war to examine a large number of anxious soldiers, my second aim is to carry a little farther some observations offered in Chapter 2. In that chapter I described in some detail the psychopathology underlying the neurotic breakdown of three military patients with previous histories which differed greatly with respect to the incidences of previous overt anxiety, offering the tentative conclusions then that the presence of anxiety symptoms, both in childhood and in adult life, is often of good prognostic significance in that individuals who had been capable of tolerating relatively great amounts of anxiety during the course of development proved on the whole less liable to develop relatively irreversible neurotic reactions in the face of traumatic war experiences.

[1] Paper read before the British Psycho-Analytical Society on 4 May 1949 and first published in the *Int. J. Psycho-Anal.* (1949), **30**.

From its earliest period, psychoanaytic theory regarding the nature of anxiety has approached the subject from two points of view. In the first place, the relationship of anxiety to instinctual frustration has often been stressed. Although Freud made considerable modifications in the conception and orientation of his hypothesis, he continued to stress the close relationship of anxiety to quantities of frustrated instinctual tension. The importance of this notion has always been generally accepted by analytical writers. Otto Fenichel (1945), for example, frequently refers to the pathogenic effect of what he calls 'dammed up' states, a term also used by Anna Freud in *The Ego and Mechanisms of Defence*, and Ernest Jones, too, has from a very early date stressed the vital significance of mounting instinctual tension for which no discharge is available as a factor in emergence of anxiety. In addition, Ernest Jones in particular has interpreted anxiety from a biological point of view, emphasizing the close relationship between anxiety and fear. As early as 1911 he explicitly stated:

> Desire that can find no direct expression is 'introverted', and the dread that arises is really the patient's dread of an outburst of his own buried desire. In other words, morbid anxiety subserves the same biological function as normal fear, in that it protects the organism against mental processes of which it is afraid (1911, p. 423).

In what may be regarded as his definitive statements on the subject in 'Inhibitions, Symptoms and Anxiety' (1926) and in the 'New Introductory Lectures' (1933) Freud similarly distinguishes between two types of anxiety. While he recognizes and explicitly states the value of anxiety as a response to an internal danger situation, he does not abandon his earlier interpretation of anxiety as the accumulation of excitation which cannot be discharged. He thus gives the name primary anxiety, or the traumatic factor, to the condition which, he states, is directly brought about by helplessness in the face of overwhelming instinctual excitation. Secondary anxiety, in contrast, he defines as a defensive reaction which becomes manifest as a signal that a danger situation may arise. Freud concluded in the 'New Introductory Lectures': 'I can see no objection to there being a twofold origin of anxiety—one as a direct consequence of the traumatic moment and the other as a signal threatening a repetition of such a moment' (1933, p. 94 f.).

ANXIETY

This chapter is based on Freud's distinction between two types of anxiety, and his definition of primary anxiety as the direct result of such helplessness in a situation of overwhelming excitation as to constitute a traumatic event. Secondary anxiety, however great, is defined as a defensive reaction brought about by fear in the face of an internal danger situation. In considering the capacity of the individual to bear anxiety, this dichotomy must be borne in mind. Instinctual excitation or tension of any kind will at some point reach a pitch sufficient to precipitate traumatic or primary anxiety. One might postulate three possible stages in this development. In the first stage, while instinctual tension remains well within the individual capacity for its toleration, it will not constitute a danger situation; rather it will be experienced as a specific tension, for example sexual desire, but without anxiety. In the second stage, the instinctual tension will have reached a pitch nearer to the breaking point of the individual so that an internal danger situation is created. At this point true anxiety of the secondary type will be experienced. Finally, after tension reaches a pitch which cannot be tolerated, either with or without intervening secondary anxiety, a traumatic event will occur, characterized by the appearance of primary anxiety.

In discussing anxiety, therefore, we have a double task: first we must consider both the origin and psychogenesis of instinctual frustration, and second we must formulate and describe the way in which this frustration presents itself as an internal danger situation. That is to say, we must first consider briefly the various views regarding the basic primary instincts and the conditions determining their frustration; secondly, we must consider the specific internal danger situations which arise in the course of mental development. In both these questions we approach controversial matters, since the part played by aggressive instincts with respect to instinctual tension and internal danger situations is a matter of considerable difference of opinion. To put the extremes of the controversy in simplest form, we must ask and answer the question: Is anxiety, either partially or wholly, produced by or in response to primary aggressive impulses; or, on the other hand, should aggression be regarded as secondary, arising either as a result of external frustration or as a direct response to anxiety itself? At one extreme, Melanie Klein (1946) and others stress the generative role of the primary aggressive or destructive impulses in anxiety. At the other, John Bowlby (1946) doubts the existence of primary aggression as an independent pathogenic factor, relating its appearance rather to external frustration of primitive instinctual impulses. Midway between these two extreme points of view Rudolph Loewenstein (1940), in a paper entitled 'The Vital or Somatic Instincts', makes a case for the reinstatement of the self-preservative instincts as primary; and Freud states in 'Inhibitions, Symptoms and Anxiety' that 'what we are concerned with are scarcely ever pure instinctual impulses but mixtures in various proportions of the two groups of instincts' (1926, p. 125). In his paper 'Psycho-Analysis and the Instincts' Ernest Jones also concludes that

> the erotizing of aggressive impulses is a remarkable general process which accounts for much of the complexity of life. For these reasons it is extraordinarily difficult to detect spontaneous activity of the aggressive instinct in isolation, and I do not myself know of any unequivocal example (1936, p. 196).

While we must forgo a full discussion of the nature of the basic instincts, it is essential to recognize that the question of the nature of the aggressive instincts is pivotal here. There would, I think, be general agreement that in respect of clinical conditions, and in the course of every analysis, anxiety can be seen either as a response to, or as a cause of, aggressive impulses which are either conscious or threatening to become so. We are all familiar, in short, with the child who becomes aggressive because he is anxious. Anna Freud has devoted a chapter to this type of aggression in *The Ego and the Mechanisms of Defence*, under the title 'Identification with the Aggressor'. Theodor Reik has published a paper under the title 'Aggression from Anxiety', in which he expanded this topic at some length, stating that: 'We have hitherto underestimated the significance of this mechanism whereby anxiety is transformed into hatred and so into aggressive tendencies' (1941, p. 9). Paula Heimann (1942) also refers to the vicious circle created by aggressiveness and anxiety, implying that each reacts with and aggravates the other.

General agreement about clinical manifestations does not, however, by any means imply any real consensus of opinion, either with regard to the existence of aggression as a primary instinct, as to whether this aggression is in the first instance directed towards the self (i.e. the 'death instinct') or towards the outside world. Nor is there agreement as to the degree and manner in which the instincts are regarded by the ego as inherently dangerous. To review the points of view held by some of the analysts who have made important statements on the subject, Melanie Klein states, in 'Schizoid Mechanisms': 'I hold that anxiety arises from the operation of the death instinct within the organism, is felt as fear of annihilation (death) and takes the form of fear of persecution' (1946, p. 296). Although in an earlier paper she has also stated that 'from the very beginning of life libido is fused with aggressiveness' (1945, p. 378), it is clear that in her opinion the ultimate source of anxiety is attributable to primary destructive impulses directed towards the ego. Anna Freud, without specifying the nature of the instincts concerned, definitely includes dread of the strength of the instincts as an important cause of deep anxiety, stating that 'if the demands of the instinctual impulses become excessive, its [the ego's] mute hostility to instinct is intensified to the point of anxiety' (1936). Ernest Jones also implies the decisive importance of instinctual danger in his paper on 'The Genesis of the Super-Ego', in which he states:

> Whether there is a separate aggressive instinct in man or not, it is certain that the sexual one is, especially in its primordial stage, essentially aggressive in its nature—far more so than psycho-analysts originally thought . . . There is good reason to suppose that these aggressive components are felt by the infant to be in themselves harmful or dangerous, quite directly so and apart from any effects on either the infant or the loved object. The response to them is anxiety, and at first what may be called pre-ideational anxiety, i.e. without any sense of the nature of the danger (1947, p. 151 f.).

To sum up, whatever one's orientation towards the basic instincts, there is no doubt that the idea that sexual and aggressive impulses which cannot be tolerated become manifest as primary anxiety, is still fruitful as a means of increasing our clinical understanding of traumatic states. It is important to realize, however, that although this conception was first expressed in relation to sexual impulses, modern developments have led to relatively greater emphasis on the part played in early anxiety states by aggressive and destructive tendencies. Since, moreover, the conception of frustration as a source of instinctual tension plays an important part in this theory, the hypothesis that aggression, tension and anxiety react in an increasing vicious circle under unfavourable circumstances can be easily correlated with this point of view.

As has been stated already, when this tension, however created, becomes intolerable, traumatic anxiety results. If this frustration is present in lesser degrees, the consequent tension is, according to Freud's conception, experienced by the individual as an internal danger situation. The biological response to danger situations, whether internal or external, is to develop fear. Secondary anxiety, thus defined as the purposive response to an internal danger situation, is a conception of the utmost importance. We are here also concerned with a subject on which many differences of opinion exist. To put the problem again in its simplest form: Assuming that instinctual frustration is the determinant of an internal danger situation, how much are we to attribute this danger situation to a frustration-promoting external environment, and how much are we to regard the frustration as something inherent in the nature of human psychological make-up? This problem is closely related to the topic just discussed—that is, the nature of the primary instincts themselves. The emphasis, however, must be somewhat different. Here we are concerned to consider the effect of internal danger situations on the individual. This should not be taken as minimizing the importance of external reality or the relationship of anxiety to external frustration or danger.

The thesis here is not so much that external events are unimportant, as that their pathogenic action lies in the internal situations brought about when accumulated instinctual frustration, however originated, reaches a pitch sufficient to constitute an internal threat. Here, too, we are concerned with important differences of opinion as to how far this instinctual frustration may be attributed to external situations, and to what degree frustrations are inevitable because the instincts themselves are essentially dangerous. As we showed earlier, the work of the modern English school is based on the premise that danger arises from the instincts themselves. It appears that Anna Freud (cf.

1936) also accepts this view. Freud himself, although accepting the conception that instinctual frustration is the determinant of an internal danger situation, implied that this situation was brought about not so much by fear of the instincts themselves, as by the possible resultant external threat, particularly that of castration. In this connection he stated explicitly in 'Inhibitions, Symptoms and Anxiety' that 'instinctual demand is, after all, not dangerous in itself; it only becomes so inasmuch as it entails a real external danger, the danger of castration' (1926, p. 126).

To make explicit the points of agreement, as well as those of disagreement: the conception of anxiety as a response to an internal danger situation, however produced, cannot be regarded as controversial within psychoanalytical circles. We have already touched on the relationship of the internal danger situation to the instincts and their frustration. Once accepted, the conception of an internal danger situation is a wide one, including not only anxiety produced in direct relation to the instincts themselves, but also anxiety arising in relation to objects. Anna Freud, for example, states quite specifically that 'The effect of the anxiety experienced by the ego because of the strength of the instincts is the same as that produced by the super-ego anxiety' (1936, p. 64). Since one internal object, the superego, is accepted as a source of anxiety, I can see no theoretical difficulty in expanding this idea to include anxiety arising from more primitive internal objects, namely the precursors of the superego. Nor in this connection should there be any difficulty in allowing the possibility that anxiety situations of different types may arise according to whether the ego feels itself directly threatened by an attacking internal object (i.e. paranoid anxiety), or whether the fear and danger are more directly related to possible loss of a good object (i.e. depressive anxiety). Both types of anxiety situation can be readily recognized as arising from external danger situations. Freud, for example, specifically distinguishes between the external danger related to possible attack in attributing phobia formation to objective fear of a castrating father, and the earlier anxiety situations in which the danger arises more directly in relation to fear of the withdrawal of a good or protecting object, namely the mother. I am suggesting, in brief, that once the possibility of these being internal precursors of the superego is accepted, the appearance of internal danger situations related to them must be accepted as inevitable.

A distinction can be made, then, between internal danger situations directly attributable to instinctual frustration as such and internal danger situations which on analysis can be interpreted as deriving from threats arising from internal objects. It will be obvious, however, that this separation, although valid, is artificial, and only justifiable for purposes of description. Although there are, as has been emphasized, considerable differences of opinion both as to the nature of the instincts concerned and as to the structure and significance of internal objects preceding the definitive and generally accepted superego, there is no difference of opinion as to the fundamental inseparability of instinct from internal object. As Freud says in the 'New Introductory Lectures':

> There is no doubt that, when the super-ego was first instituted, in equipping that agency use was made of the piece of the child's aggressiveness towards his parents for which he was unable to effect a discharge outwards . . .; and for that reason the severity of the super-ego need not simply correspond to the strictness of the upbringing. It is very possible that, when there are later occasions for suppressing aggressiveness, the instinct may take the same path that was opened to it at that decisive point of time. . . .
>
> Theoretically we are in fact in doubt whether we should suppose that all the aggressiveness that has returned from the external world is bound by the super-ego and accordingly turned against the ego, or that a part of it is carrying on its mute and uncanny activity as a free destructive instinct in the ego and the id. A distribution of the latter kind is the more probable; but we know nothing more about it (1933, p. 109).

These statements not only make clear the apparent inseparability of instinct from object, but also still leave open the theoretical possibility that unbound destructive instinct may remain a potential source of internal danger situations. Melanie Klein, in 'Schizoid Mechanisms', shows that in her opinion, too, instincts and internal objects can be separated only in descriptive theoretical terms, since

> The fear of the destructive impulse seems to attach itself at once to an object—or rather it is experienced as fear of an uncontrollable, overpowering object. . . . Even if these objects are felt to be external, they become through introjection internal persecutors and thus reinforce the fear of the destructive impulse within (1946, p. 296).

I should like to digress for a moment here to raise another point. I have not, so far, attempted to make any distinction between conscious and unconscious anxiety. The concept of unconscious anxiety presents a number of theoretical difficulties, although a great deal of analytical theory is based on its existence. In considering this problem it is important to specify the type of anxiety under discussion. With regard to primary anxiety it is difficult to be precise. In those situations which have been described as traumatic the physical and mental manifestations obviously affect the whole of mental and physical life. Such events are, for example, the infant at birth and in other situations of total helplessness in the face of overwhelming excitation, and the adult when this situation is repeated in a traumatic experience. When instinctual tension of this type is present in intolerable quantities, it may be guarded against by a number of different defences. Accumulation of inner tension has been defined as the determinant of the internal situation to which secondary anxiety is the purposive biological response. Since it is associated with the mental and physical changes which are the inevitable accompaniment of fear in any danger situation, external or internal, secondary anxiety so defined will, when it is developed and tolerated as such, produce conscious manifestations. There may be, however, a number of other defences against this threatened internal danger situation which either prevent the emergence of, or disguise the subjective experience of, true secondary anxiety with full awareness of its mental and physical aspects.

My contention is that the development and toleration of secondary anxiety may be not only inevitable, but also desirable as a stimulus to early infantile development, and as an essential prerequisite for the construction of adequate defences in all danger situations, whether they arise from within or from without. The physical and mental manifestations of this type of anxiety are closely related to the physical and mental accompaniments of normal fear, i.e. fear which prepares the individual for action in an objective or external danger situation. According to most accepted physiological and psychological theories, the physical and mental changes developed in this situation are unequivocally purposive in that they prepare the individual to deal with a threatened danger. Psychologically, that is to say, the anxious individual will be conscious of some feeling of anticipatory dread, mental alertness, and tension. Physically he will produce some or all of those physical changes which in an external danger situation would equip him either to fight or to take flight. A good example of the stimulating effects of this type of anxiety in a real-life situation which we must all have experienced is that of impending examinations. This situation can also be used to illustrate the difference between anxiety as a stimulating and as an inhibiting factor. When anxiety retains the quality of normal purposive fear, the examinee, although subject to some uncomfortable physical sensations, is usually aware of unusual mental alertness, ability to use his resources to the best of his power, and moreover to sense and avoid the traps presented to him by a wily examiner. When, in contrast, for any reason anxiety loses these qualities and resembles rather the helpless manifestations of the infant confronted by a situation with which he cannot cope, the mind goes blank, the individual becomes tremulous and distressed, and is unable to use his resources in any purposive way.

When we try to disentangle the psychopathological differences between these two reactions, we are faced with a number of difficulties. Although the examination situation does not present an actual objective threat to the individual, it must nevertheless be regarded as a real danger in that failure entails real disadvantages. About the individual differences responsible for bringing about these different reactions to the examination situation, there has been considerable analytical literature which was summarized in a paper published by Professor Flügel (1939). Although in his paper a number of interesting interpretations of the examination situation are given, the emergence of the type of primary anxiety I have mentioned is not stressed. I feel, however, that the distinction between the incidence of primary and secondary anxiety is particularly clear in the examination situation. In the first group the danger situation is recognized and accepted as a challenge which can be prepared for and coped with, so that anxiety acts as an ally; in the second group the tension and excitation produced, far from helping, inhibit the individual and prevent him from coping with the situation. In the successful individual, it might be argued that these manifestations should not be described as due to anxiety so much as to normal fear. I use the example, however, as an illustration of the stimulating effects of fear in a danger situation—effects which I believe to be qualitatively analogous to secondary anxiety developed in response to internal unconscious danger situations.

Between the type of anxiety or fear which is entirely successful in its stimulating effects and the type of anxiety which is entirely inhibiting there is a wide range of conditions which comprise the various types of clinical anxiety, and the defences against them. To exemplify: if we assume that the optimum which we describe as normal fear produced only an amount of anxiety sufficient to act as stimulus without causing any significant subjective distress, we must next consider the individual who, although he develops more anxiety than he can deal with comfortably, is nevertheless able to tolerate this as anxiety, without being overwhelmed, without developing incapacitating physical symptoms, and without developing an examination phobia. Next we must consider the type of individual who in association with a degree of anxiety greater than the optimum readily expresses his anxiety in the form of somatic symptoms. This type of candidate will at the mild end of the scale only be aware of symptoms such as palpitations, frequency of micturition, dryness of the mouth, and the like, while at the more severe end of the scale, he may produce sufficient physical symptoms to interfere with his success. Finally we must consider the individual who, because of the degree of anxiety aroused by the thought of an examination, develops an examination phobia.

This same range may be invoked in characterizing the various responses to internal danger situations which stimulate anxiety related to unconscious sources. At the one extreme we have individuals who are able to tolerate considerable anxiety as such, when the danger situation is one which must be recognized and when no positive defences are available at the time. Next we have the important group of individuals who, although they retain the subjective awareness of a danger situation, are not able to contain this danger situation within themselves (i.e. to recognize the danger as arising from within) but who project it on to the external world in the form of a phobia. It is important to stress the fact that this group of individuals, although they manage to avoid the subjective experience of very great quantities of what Freud has described as free-floating or unspecific anxiety, nevertheless do not deny their awareness of a danger situation in spite of the fact that they project the internal danger on to the outside world.

Next in this range of diminishing awareness of internal danger situations, we have the group of individuals in whom the physical responses to anxiety play a more considerable part than the mental. These individuals are much less aware of fear than of its bodily concomitants. To consider this problem in detail would obviously take us far afield, since it involves the whole question of bodily compliance, the way in which different organs can take on special psychological significance and the way in which bodily changes at first produced by anxiety may be perpetuated, or disguised, by hysterical mechanisms. The degree and manner in which the total manifestations of anxiety, both physical and mental, may be assigned by the ego's defensive agencies are obviously of considerable interest. Gregory Zilboorg (1933), for example, in a paper entitled 'Anxiety Without Affect', has described an interesting case in which a patient produced the physical manifestations of an acute anxiety attack without emotional concomitants. Usually, dissociated physical manifestations of anxiety are more chronic in nature; it is well recognized that a person who tolerates considerable quantities of anxiety in its physical manifestations over a long period, often tends to be predisposed, either as a result of cumulative stress or of some new situation which quantitatively increases tension, to develop one of the organic diseases which are recognized to be psychosomatic in origin. Of these people Sir Heneage Ogilvie has said in the Beyer Memorial Lecture,

> In the less stoutly built, it is the mind itself that gives way. In the more stable, the mind remains coherent and calm and the mechanism working beneath it cracks under the strain. The primitive tribal emotions . . . take charge. The automatic and endocrine arsenals pour out their munitions to excess . . . (1949).

Not infrequently, the individual who develops psychosomatic disorders denies much awareness of conscious fear. Unlike phobic patients, he does not retain an awareness of a danger situation, even though he may experience many of the bodily concomitants of fear. During the war, for example, many patients of the effort syndrome type denied any experience of the emotions of fear or anxiety. This group passes by imperceptible shades into the last group, those individuals who have successfully avoided any awareness of fear or anxiety, denying the existence of danger situations, both external and internal. Individuals of this group, at the point when instinctual tension reaches a degree sufficient to constitute an internal threat, successfully deny or repress awareness of the danger situation. Unlike the other groups I have described, therefore, these individuals neither develop and tolerate anxiety—even partially or in disguised form—as do patients suffering from psychosomatic disorders; nor, on the other hand, do they acknowledge by phobic symptom formation their awareness of threatened danger situations, whether external or internal.

This point may be illustrated by a study I made in 1942 of a group of patients characterized by an apparent personality change after one specific terrifying war experience. The previous personalities of these patients all showed certain features in that they all tended to have experienced little, if any, conscious anxiety. The patients of this group could not, however, be regarded as typical of the counterphobic group described by Otto Fenichel (1939), nor had the previous personality structure apparently been grossly abnormal. In one case of this type there was every evidence to suggest that, both with regard to sexual life and with regard to capacity for sublimation, the patient had been notably well adjusted prior to his breakdown. In these cases, the individual concerned had had no previous breakdown and had often experienced severe enemy action for an appreciable length of time without developing symptoms. He had not been aware of any change in his condition up to the time of the traumatic incident. In each case the traumatic incident consisted of a terrifying experience which had the specific quality of involving some undeniable physical threat. A London fireman, who had been on fire-fighting duties during all the worst London fires, suddenly developed acute and inhibiting anxiety symptoms after receiving a very slight injury to his hand when a falling beam in a burning building touched him. Others gave similar histories. The striking thing about this group of patients, however, was that the course of recovery after the traumatic experience differed from that of the more typical war neuroses. These men did not work through their traumatic experiences by anxiety dreams, nor did they remain conspicuously anxious. Instead, after a rather quick initial recovery, they became resentful, depressed, somewhat paranoid and markedly hypochondriacal. They tended to look back at their former personalities and general health with a sense of mourning and grievance. They also showed a striking bewilderment about their symptoms, which were coloured throughout by a subjective change, both in respect of themselves and of the outside world. Even after considerable treatment this type of patient did not make a full recovery. It appeared that the change brought about by the unfamiliar and totally unprepared-for experience of severe fear or panic was more or less irreversible.

It was these men who in the first place brought to my attention the prophylactic value of previous anxiety for relatively irreversible reactions of this type, following frightening war experiences. Other groups—namely those who had shown evidence of free-floating anxiety, psychosomatic symptoms, or phobic anxiety—frequently broke down with severe symptoms following battle experience. Significantly, however, that happened only after prolonged stress sufficient to exhaust the whole individual and to reduce his capacity for enduring instinctual tension and /or the accumulation of overwhelming quantities of excitation resulting from the emergence of demonstrable primary anxiety. Even then, the tendency towards spontaneous recovery was more in evidence. In fact, the clinical picture presented by patients giving a history of previous anxiety was usually a quantitative increase in their previous symptoms unaccompanied by any marked qualitative personality change. In Chapter 2 I described one such case and stressed not only the previous evidence of phobic formation in his character, but also the fact that the specific traumatic experience leading to his breakdown was similar in every respect to the type of experience which I have described here. It was, that is to say, an experience which reactivated obvious castration fears.

During the course of the war I saw a number of other patients who showed a similar psychopathology which evoked no persistent subjective changes, and who frequently recovered to a sufficient degree to return to full military duty. For those patients who developed relatively irreversible internal changes of a regressive type, the failure to develop and cope with secondary anxiety related to unconscious castration fears appears to have been of decisive importance. Since, moreover, it is generally agreed that castration fears are integrally bound up with instinctual urges, both libidinal towards the mother and aggressive towards the father, it is evident that these patients' omnipotent denial of external danger was determined by their relative inability to tolerate the instinctual conflicts involved in the genital oedipal situation. This relative intolerance was demonstrated by manifest depression, tension and inability to cope with the changed internal situation resulting from a traumatic experience, which made untenable the previous mechanism of projecting an internal danger situation to the outside world and then denying it.

The fact that war experiences of an identical unconscious significance produced such different clinical results in these groups of patients illustrates the complex problem with which we are faced in considering the problem of anxiety. As I have suggested, we are confronted with two questions: the capacity of the organism to tolerate instinctual frustration and, secondly, the capacity of the ego to recognize, tolerate and deal with the threatened internal danger situation arising as frustration increases. At this point we must again ask ourselves the relationship between these two problems. Throughout analytical literature there is an implied contrast between manifestations of anxiety which serve positive purposes and those which take inhibiting, paralysing forms. Between the extremes lies the types of clinical condition usually considered under the heading 'anxiety states' in which, although the anxiety retains the quality of a defensive reaction, either the quantity of the anxiety or the type of defence used by the individual results in relative distress. It seems, therefore, impossible to draw a sharp distinction between useful and useless anxiety.

It may nonetheless be possible to distinguish among three gradations; there is, first, anxiety tolerated as such during critical periods of development until positive modes of defence become available. Under optimum conditions this purposive anxiety is characterized by the stimulating qualities of normal fear, but should nevertheless be defined as anxiety, since the danger situation is predominantly internal and unconscious. Secondly, there are those in whom the anxiety reaches a degree, or is dealt with by a type of defence, which must be regarded as pathological but which does serve a useful purpose in so far as these manifestations of anxiety, either phobic or psychosomatic, are preferable to the disaster against which they are erected as a defence. As both the instinctual tension constituting the danger situation and the secondary anxiety thereby stimulated increase towards the limit of individual tolerance, the purposive quality of the anxiety becomes to a greater or lesser degree overshadowed by the impending disaster. The anxiety, that is to say, becomes progressively less effectively purposive, comes more to resemble the inhibition of a panic situation. Finally, there is the situation in which the defences have broken down and the individual has become helpless in the face of overwhelming excitation. This traumatic experience represents a psychic disaster brought about by a type of anxiety manifestation not only quantitatively, but qualitatively different from the other groups. This qualitative difference is demonstrated not only by the inhibiting, paralysing nature of the acute symptomatology, in this particular group, but also by the regressive after-effects indicated by development and persistence of depression, hypochondriasis and mild paranoid tendencies—symptoms, in brief, more aptly described as produced by the reaction to a disaster than as a defensive measure against a threat.

The significance of trauma in this sense, as the disaster against which anxiety is erected, is hinted at throughout analytical literature. Freud considered the prototype of this traumatic experience to be the situation at birth, and thus developed the conception of primary anxiety underlying the present discussion. The relationship of birth to specific subsequent anxiety symptoms has also been discussed by Phyllis Greenacre (1941, 1945). Otto Fenichel also frequently refers to the pathogenic effect of dammed up states which he describes in very similar terms, contrasting this type of helplessness with purposive fear. Theodor Reik (1941), in dealing with the same qualitative differences, suggested that the terms 'fright' and 'anxiety' might be utilized. Ernest Jones, although he has always maintained that even primary anxiety is a defensive mechanism in considering the deepest sources of anxiety, nevertheless relates this anxiety to overwhelming excitation and describes its final result by stating that

> If the conception put forward here is valid we reach the conclusion that what the infant finds so intolerable in the primal 'traumatic' situation, the danger against which it feels so helpless is the loss of control in respect of libidinal excitation, its capacity to relieve it and enjoy the relief of it. If the situation is not yet allayed it can only end in the exhaustion of a temporary aphanisis, one which doubtless signifies a permanent one to the infant. All the complicated measures of defence that compose the material of our study in psycho-analysis are fundamentally endeavours to avoid this consummation (1929, p. 315).

It appears that Jones attributes this state mainly to loss of control of libidinal excitation, whereas Melanie Klein would likely attribute traumatic or primary anxiety of this type to a situation in which the ego felt itself temporarily overwhelmed by the destructive instinct. Nevertheless, in spite of differences of opinion, analysts of every theoretical orientation would agree that the traumatic experience is closely related to helplessness in a situation of overwhelming excitation in which the individual not only feels abandoned by all good objects, but facing attack and extermination by all bad ones, be they external or internal.

I have described some clinical evidence which suggested that the failure to develop anxiety seen in these patients, although related at a genital level to denial of castration fear, was ultimately determined by the previously denied recognition of this original danger situation with the result that once danger became inescapable, regression to the earliest level became inevitable. This implied argument to the effect that secondary anxiety is indispensable, both as an aid towards development and as a protection against psychic disaster, may at first sight appear paradoxical except to those who agree with Melanie Klein's statement to the effect that 'the very anxiety which is pre-eminently an inhibiting agency in the development of the individual is also a factor of fundamental importance in promoting growth of his ego' (1932). I am suggesting that whatever one's orientation towards the basic instincts, and whatever the relative emphasis laid on external and internal factors, danger situations in infancy will nevertheless first appear in relation to instinctual tension and frustration, i.e. in relation to an internal situation. Danger situations so determined are, in my opinion, inevitable even under optimal external conditions, and however well they may be dealt with by the various mechanisms at our disposal, cannot be eliminated as potential sources of further danger. The conflicts which have determined these danger situations remain buried in the deepest levels of the unconscious from the cradle to the grave, so that under unfavourable conditions, either externally or internally determined, they may be revived at any period of life. Secondary anxiety, defined as the appropriate biological response to these internal danger situations, is thus indispensable at every stage of development.

Not only, moreover, do I believe that the capacity to develop and tolerate secondary anxiety is decisive in the achievement of mental stability and health, but also I should like to suggest that this capacity is important to an allied subject of vital clinical significance: the limitations of analysis as a therapeutic process. In this connection, the dichotomy I have been stressing throughout is also apparent. With regard to the capacity to tolerate instinctual frustration, I should like to quote Ernest Jones' remarks in his valedictory address:

> There may well be an innate factor akin to the General Intelligence G, the nature of which it still remains to elucidate, but which may be of cardinal importance in the final endeavour to master the deepest infantile anxieties, to tolerate painful ego-dystonic impulses or affects, and so to attain the balanced mentality that is our ideal. It has occurred to me further that if such a factor can ever be isolated it may prove to have a physiological basis which will bring us back to the often neglected problems of heredity. The capacity to endure the non-gratification of a wish without either reacting to the privation or renouncing the wish, holding it as it were in suspense, probably corresponds with a neurological capacity, perhaps of an electrical nature, to retain the stimulating effects of an afferent impulse without immediately discharging them in an efferent direction (1946, p. 10).

I believe that further research into this question may well

indicate limits for analysis in treatment of personality problems, borderline cases and psychotics. It may be that patients who tend to develop anxiety with the inhibiting qualities of the primary type whenever tension increases have not only been so hampered from the dawn of life as to have failed to reach a level of ego development at which secondary anxiety was developed, but also tend in the analytic situation to repeat this traumatic experience with manifestations such as to raise considerable doubt as to their capacity for ultimate satisfactory development. Although this point is certainly controversial, most analysts would probably agree that it is this quality of the potential psychotic which makes analysis outside of an institution so difficult. The general hypothesis seems to me compatible with other analytical theories regarding the predisposition to psychosis, theories which stress, from a somewhat different point of view, the intensity and intolerability of the deep anxiety underlying psychotic conflicts. I wish to underline what I believe to be the qualitative difference between two types of anxiety, emphasizing the failure of the psychotic to develop or tolerate stimulating or purposive anxiety of the secondary type. Gregory Zilboorg (1933) has also hinted at the possible close relationship between psychotic and primary anxiety, suggesting that the physical tension, perplexity and distress preceding psychotic regression may also represent a repetition of the birth trauma.

For neurotics the capacity to recognize and tolerate the existence of an internal, unconsciously determined danger situation by developing secondary anxiety is decisive. This capacity is very closely linked to the problem of psychological insight. If anxiety is defined as the response to an internal danger situation, the capacity to develop and tolerate anxiety, associated as it must always be with an unconscious conflict, is very closely related to the capacity to recognize and tolerate the instinctual conflicts and tension which constitute the threatened internal danger situation. This means that the more an individual has been able, in an internal, unconsciously produced danger situation, to develop and tolerate anxiety, the more one finds in analysis that he is capable of facing and resolving the conflict which determined it. Conversely, the more the individual has tended to defend himself against anxiety, by the development of hysterical symptoms, severe psychosomatic symptoms, or by the omnipotent denial of danger, the less will he be capable of tolerating insight in its literal sense of looking within. In the analysis of neurotic patients, this capacity for achieving and tolerating the anxiety associated with insight is of decisive importance.

To conclude, this chapter recapitulates briefly the historical development of analytical theories regarding the nature of anxiety, stressing the importance of the distinction between primary and secondary anxiety. To some extent this has involved oversimplification of this distinction which, as will be obvious, is not by any means always so sharp or so clear as the argument would suggest. Omitted has been a discussion of the closely related problems of the tolerance of guilt and depression. Nevertheless, it seems that the distinction between anxiety as a psychic disaster resulting from something which has not been tolerated, and anxiety as the purposive response to a threatened danger which has not yet taken place is valid, and that it throws considerable light on many clinical problems. It has been suggested that two factors are essential for successful development. First, there must be capacity to endure instinctual tension sufficient to allow the threat of a traumatic situation to develop, and secondly, there must be an ability to recognize this threat by developing anxiety of the purposive, biological type, which may be utilized as a means of securing and maintaining satisfactory development and mental health.

4

DEPRESSIVE ILLNESS[1]

(1960)

Depression, like anxiety, is a universal subjective experience integral to human development and the mastery of conflict, frustration, disappointment and loss. At the same time, however, depression, again like anxiety, is not only to be regarded as an affective experience of general psychological significance; it is also the main presenting symptom of a regressive clinical syndrome as severe, characteristic and well defined as any to be found in the whole field of clinical psychiatry. This illness, moreover, because of its frequent occurrence in patients with a positive family history and its association with specific periods of biological significance, poses crucial problems as to the relation between psychogenic, environmental and constitutional factors in the development and structure of mental illness.

To begin at a familiar point of departure, Karl Abraham, pioneer in this field, emphasized the role of constitutional factors in depressive illness. He also indicated the general significance of depression as a symptom which might be compared and contrasted with anxiety. 'The affect of depression', he said in 1911, 'is as widely spread among all forms of neuroses and psychoses as is that of anxiety. . . . Anxiety and depression are related to each other in the same way as are fear and grief. We fear a coming evil; we grieve over one that has occurred' (p. 137). Certain aspects of recent psychoanalytic theory might be epitomized by comparing with Abraham's a statement from Edward Bibring's 1953 paper, 'The Mechanism of Depression'. 'Anxiety and depression', says Bibring,

> represent diametrically opposed basic ego responses. Anxiety as a reaction to . . . danger indicates the ego's desire to survive. The ego, challenged by the danger, mobilizes the signal of anxiety and

[1] Paper read at the 21st Congress of the International Psycho-Analytical Association, Copenhagen, in July 1959. First published in the *Int. J. Psycho-Anal.* (1960), **41**.

prepares for fight or flight. In depression, the opposite takes place; the ego is paralysed because it finds itself incapable to meet the 'danger' (1953, p. 34 f.).

The key word, of course, in this more recent formulation is 'ego'. Freud's initial concept of anxiety maintained a theoretical distinction between fear and anxiety which delayed recognition of the role of anxiety as the stimulus for adaptive defences. While his later formulations enriched our understanding of the central role of anxiety in psychic development, difficult problems remained for the theoretical definition of pathological anxiety states. Parallel and related considerations apply to the distinction between depression as a general affective experience and depressive illness as a complex regressive syndrome. Abraham, for example, suggested that depression, like anxiety, might be attributable to repression. 'We can distinguish', he said, 'between the affect of sadness or grief and neurotic depression, the latter being unconsciously motivated and a consequence of repression' (1911, p. 137). Bibring's concept of depression as a basic ego response, though in some respects controversial, emphasized the crucial importance of depression as an affect integral to psychic life. At the same time, however, this general concept of depression does not answer many questions relevant to the structure and meanings of pathological depression, particularly depressive illness.

While our concepts of anxiety and depression as affects with general psychological significance have thus changed with the development of ego psychology, Abraham's original formulations with regard to depressive illness appear over the passage of time to have become more, rather than less, compatible with the general body of psychoanalytic knowledge. In particular, the importance he attached to object relations, aggression and the mastery of ambivalence has been confirmed by psychoanalysts of every school. In both his 1911 paper and in his more extensive 1924 monograph, Abraham approached the developmental, theoretical interpretation of depressive illness via a detailed and perceptive understanding of its clinical phenomenology. The patients whose psychopathology he discussed were beyond any reasonable question depressed. Subsequent psychoanalytic discussions of depression have, in contrast, frequently been obscured by two factors: first, failure clearly to distinguish depression as a symptom which may arise in the widest variety of clinical conditions ranging from normal grief to overt schizophrenic disorder, from depressive illness as a specific psychiatric syndrome; and, second, emphasis on infantile precursors to the relative neglect of definitive adult psychopathology.

The relation of early experience to adult pathology is, of course, a crucial problem for the psychoanalytic understanding of mental illness. The continued activity of primitive unresolved conflicts in adult mental disorder remains a fundamental corollary of the dynamic approach to mental life. A number of psychoanalytic formulations have focused primarily on suggested similarities between adult symptomatology and reconstructed early experiences. Freud's proposals concerning the nature of major hysterical attacks and Otto Rank's theory of the birth trauma (1924) are classical examples of this type of psychoanalytic reconstruction. The archaic features of overt depressive illness lend themselves to a similar approach. Abraham, Radó, Klein, Jacobson and others have attempted to understand adult depression by reconstructing its infantile prototype. Abraham suggested the hypothesis, subsequently elaborated and expanded by Jacobson, that disappointment at the oedipal level reinforced or regressively revived unresolved pregenital conflicts, resulting in repetitive depressive responses to subsequent disappointment and loss. Radó drew analogies between the infant's nursing experiences and the depressed ego's attitude towards its own superego.

The most far-reaching analogies between adult depressive illness and early developmental phases have been proposed by Melanie Klein and the English school. They have postulated a universal infantile depressive position the general characteristics of which determine depressive responses in adult life. The primary importance attached to early object relations in this context converges in certain respects with hypotheses put forward by psychoanalysts of very different orientation—there is considerable consensus as to the relevance of early experience to the predisposition of depression. A crucial question, however, concerns the degree to which regressive symptomatology in adult life represents a direct repetition of the original developmental process. Melanie Klein, although she has explicitly stated that her hypothesis does not imply overt clinical depression in infancy, clearly suggests that the unconscious struggles and fantasies characteristic of the infant's mental life are revived in the dreams, fantasies and affective experiences of the adult depressive patient. Similarities between adult depressive illness and early responses to real or threatened object loss are also integral to otherwise very different reconstructions proposed by Abraham, Jacobson, Radó and Spitz. The common premise underlying these theories is that adult depressive illness closely resembles an infantile prototype.

Stimulating and important though such reconstructive efforts may be, they tend to raise questions similar to those aroused by Otto Rank's theory of the birth trauma as the definitive explanation of pathological anxiety. While in this context recent work, in particular that of Phyllis Greenacre, confirms the potential pathogenic implications of birth and the early postnatal period, a crucial distinction has been proposed between infantile experiences leading to predisposition, and understanding of the specific content or meaning of a definitive clinical syndrome in adult life. A similar approach in recent analytic thought concerns the relation between infantile problems in establishing and maintaining satisfactory object relations and overt depressive illness in adult life. In contrast, however, to those who stress infantile prototypes of adult depression, others (Bowlby, Rank, Mahler, Rochlin) emphasize the significance of early disturbances as potential factors in developmental failure, often leading to poor object relations and lack of capacity for sadness and grief. Gregory Rochlin doubts the capacity of the infant and young child to develop genuine depression and suggests that depressive illness can only develop in a relatively mature individual. Others, although they do not take such an extreme view, nevertheless emphasize the primary importance of early experience in determining ego development and the capacity for genuine object relations. While traumatic experiences in this area may be integrally related to the predisposition to depressive illness, this does not necessarily imply that adult depression is to be regarded as the direct repetition of early experience.

Freud himself was of course explicit in his recognition that, however close the dynamic similarities between early pregenital conflicts and their regressive revival in adult illness, specific content is inevitably determined by the level from which regression has taken place. The importance, moreover, of certain life situations in determining the emergence of psychic illness has always been recognized. In general, however, the psychoanalytic developmental hypothesis has been interpreted until very recently as implying, first, that adult symptomatology directly repeats infantile experience, and second, that psychic development is in many respects complete by the beginning of the latency period. Gregory Rochlin's suggestion that true depressive illness can only develop in relative maturity, however controversial, indicates an expansion of the developmental hypothesis implicit in much recent analytic writing and research. Widespread recognition of the importance of adolescence as a developmental phase may be cited as the classical example of this expansion of the developmental hypothesis. Grete Bibring and her colleagues have studied childbirth considered as a normal developmental crisis. Therese Benedek has proposed a similar hypothesis not only in respect of childbirth, but also in relation to the menopause. Kurt Eissler has investigated patients faced with imminent death, and the very word 'geriatrics' indicates increased interest in the problems of old age. The most ambitious and far-reaching suggestions in this area have been formulated by Erik Erikson in a number of stimulating contributions in which he delineates a series of developmental stages. His concepts have been incorporated in recent metapsychological proposals formulated by David Rapaport and Merton Gill, in which the adaptive hypothesis is for the first time defined as a metapsychological assumption (1959).

Freud's definitive formulations on anxiety clearly foreshadowed this expansion of the developmental hypothesis. 'Each situation of danger', he said, 'corresponds to a particular period of life or a particular developmental phase of the mental apparatus and appears to be justifiable for it' (1926, p. 146). With the development of ego psychology and the related increase in recognition of the ego's adaptive functions initiated by Hartmann's work, the developmental hypothesis has expanded in two ways. First, by the introduction of a developmental approach to the ego itself; second, by recognition of the fact that not only childhood, but the whole life cycle, must be understood in a developmental approach to the theory of depressive illness. From the outset psychoanalysts have recognized the importance of innate constitutional and biological factors in the development of depressive illness. This is an illness the relative frequency of which in adolescence, after childbirth, and in the involutional period must be explained. Moreover, the role of precipitating external events of obvious time-related significance, such as graduation, retirement, separation and object loss, points to the importance of environmental factors. This expansion of the developmental hypothesis may facilitate understanding of the frustrations and challenges characteristic of different periods of life. It must, however, be emphasized that such an approach does not imply diminished emphasis on the crucial importance of the earliest years. Erikson's concept of basic trust, for example, should be cited in this context as only one instance of the increased importance attached in our current analytic contributions to the early mother–child relationship. A new dimension, rather, has been added, at least implicitly—time. In addition to asking why an individual develops depressive illness, which may well be determined in the early years, we should now ask, in a developmental context, an additional question: when? At what period of life and under what circumstances has a depressive illness developed? In this way we may be able to understand how both dynamic and economic changes related to biological factors and events in the external world which influence object relations may determine the genesis, development and resolution of depressive illness.

A central problem in speaking of these developmental phases concerns the structure and function of the ego. Freud proposed a dualistic theory to distinguish between primary anxiety or a traumatic situation in which the ego is helpless, and secondary or 'signal' anxiety as the response of a relatively mature ego to an internal danger. On the one hand, expansion of the developmental approach requires elucidation of the specific internal dangers characteristic of different periods of life. On the other hand, a qualitative differentiation is here implied between anxiety which acts primarily as the stimulus for defensive adaptive efforts, and anxiety in which the ego either because of immaturity or because of regressive modification is flooded by stimuli it cannot master. The relationship of the latter sort of anxiety to Edward Bibring's ego-psychological approach to depression is highly significant. We must, however, make a distinction between the total helplessness implied by Freud's definition of a traumatic situation and the relative helplessness implicit in Bibring's conception of loss of self-esteem, which may indeed be compared with Freud's signal theory of anxiety.

Discussions of clinical anxiety have attempted to elucidate the complicated interrelationship between the two kinds of anxiety postulated by Freud. The fact that, as Max Schur has suggested, the ego itself may under certain conditions regress in the face of internal danger is of decisive importance in determining both the quantity and the quality of anxiety. A distinction may thus be proposed between anxiety which essentially retains its signal functions without significant regressive modification of the ego, and more pathological anxiety in which such modification takes place. An ego-psychological approach to depression facilitates a similar differentiation, within a unified conceptual framework, between normal or neurotic depression and overt depressive illness. It may be suggested that in so far as clinical depression is confined to a sense of inadequacy and transient loss of self-esteem, we are dealing with a symptom within the range of normal or neurotic experience. By contrast, depressive illness, like incapacitating anxiety states, involves more complex regressive changes. It is not only that the ego suffers a loss of self-esteem but also that this experience initiates far-reaching changes within the psychic apparatus as a whole. The ego of the seriously depressed patient has undergone qualitative regressive alterations with associated intrapsychic changes of a widespread nature. The relation, however, between regression as a loss of mature ego functions with the emergence of primitive archaic mechanisms—in both anxiety and depression—and the original process of development and maturation remains an area of considerable obscurity and controversy.

The changes themselves are less controversial than their relation to infantile precursors. There are indeed broad areas of agreement with respect to the dynamic, economic and structural characteristics, both of the predisposed individual and of depressive illness itself. For example, the specific vulnerability of the depression-prone individual to disappointment, frustration and loss is generally recognized. Sándor Radó, in his classical paper (1928), described characteristics which resemble in all essentials those which Sacha Nacht emphasizes (1960). These general predisposing characteristics have been described in terms differing according as the theoretical position of contributors differs. The need, however, for unqualified love (i.e. narcissistic supplies) and the relation of this need to unmastered aggression is generally accepted as an indication of the importance of insecure, ambivalent object relations as a predisposing cause of serious depressive responses to loss and frustration. There remains, of course, a wide range of theoretical approaches to the nature and significance of the aggressive instinct. The crucial importance of unmastered aggression in the theory of depressive illness may, however, be summarized by comparing once more a statement from Karl Abraham's original description (1911) with Edward Bibring's more recent formulation (1953). 'In every one of these cases', said Abraham, 'it could be discovered that the disease proceeded from an attitude of hate which was paralysing the patient's capacity to love. ... The pronounced feelings of inadequacy from which such patients suffer arise from this discomforting internal perception' (pp. 143, 145). 'The blow to self-esteem', said Bibring, 'is due to the unexpected awareness of the existence of latent aggressive tendencies within the self, with all the consequences involved' (p. 25).

Both Freud and Abraham recognized that the withdrawal from the outside world and from real objects so characteristic of depressive illness involves complex internalizations as a result of which the depressed patient's unmastered aggression is directed against his own ego by a hostile, recriminative superego. There is also an ego identification with the negative devalued aspects of the lost object. While these original constructions retain a high degree of validity, subsequent writers have differed both in their formulations of the mechanisms involved and in their reconstructions of the developmental process, especially those concerning the origin and structure of the superego. Some have stressed in this connection the significance of identification as an ego–superego mechanism. Others, like Abraham and Melanie Klein, emphasize the mode of instinctual activity, in particular oral incorporation and the related mechanism of introjection. As David Rapaport has indicated, the relation between these internalizing processes remains difficult and obscure. That they are crucial for depression and that regressive modifications of both ego and superego result is, on the whole, generally accepted.

Related to this difficult and obscure area is the whole problem of the regressive implications of depressive illness. There is first of all the need to differentiate between characteristics of the predisposed individual which suggest developmental failure and those which suggest significant regression during the course of illness. It is here that current psychoanalysis appears to differ most widely from early formulations. In emphasizing both its oral and its anal significance, Abraham's was primarily an attempt to understand the symptomatology of depressive illness in terms of its unconscious content of meaning. No one who has treated a seriously depressed patient can fail to confirm the validity of his observations. Whereas, however, Abraham regarded depressive illness primarily as the result of instinctual regression to a level of pregenital fantasy, we would tend today to focus primarily on the regressive modifications of both ego and superego which facilitate the emergence of primitive and archaic fantasy. While the vulnerability of the individual ego may be largely determined by the experiences of early developmental failings, this by no means implies that instinctual regression is the primary determining factor for depressive illness.

The current relevance of Abraham's comparison of depression and anxiety suggests that in certain respects psychoanalytic theory has come the full orbit—back to its original point of departure. The orbit itself, however, must now be approached from a new angle. Depression, like anxiety, is integral to human development and experience. While anxiety may be defined as the ego's response to a disaster which threatens, depression represents its response to one which has materialized. Both responses range from a mild signal to a devastating pathological syndrome. As the signal fails to elicit adaptive responses the ego itself is regressively changed. Predisposition to manifest depressive illness is probably determined at an early stage of ego development. Failure to establish and to maintain positive ego identifications based on good object relations, however determined and however conceptualized, substantially impairs both ego and superego development. Related ambivalence and unmastered aggression render the individual vulnerable to disappointment and frustration in adult life. Analytic theories concerning the relation that specific fantasies, experiences and affects characteristic of early developmental phases have to adult symptomatology are widely divergent. Differences of opinion and differences of terminology should not, however, blind us to the substantial areas of essential agreement as to the dynamic, structural and economic significance of depressive illness itself. Expansion of the developmental hypothesis may lead to increased understanding of the depressive potentialities of succeeding stages of the life cycle. The fundamental blueprints, however, for the psychoanalytic understanding of depressive illness were drawn with amazing accuracy by Freud and by Abraham in their classical papers on this subject.

5

THE DEPRESSIVE POSITION[1]

(1953)

It is well known that the most significant feature of Melanie Klein's work is her attempt to explore and analyse the mental life of the very young infant. The theoretical framework within which her concept of the 'depressive position' has developed, and with which I am mainly concerned in this chapter, rests on certain premises about this early preverbal period. These premises are controversial in many respects. In the first place Melanie Klein (1932, 1948) and most of her followers believe that, almost from birth and independent of external experience, the infant has innate unconscious knowledge concerning the differences between the sexes and the relationship between the parents. This unconscious knowledge, she suggests, gives rise to a complex fantasy life which plays a decisive role in early development. Melanie Klein also postulates, and in fact bases many of her most important theories on, the existence of a primary death instinct which is from the outset directed against the self. It is her contention, too, that processes of introjection and projection constitute the basic mental mechanisms of the first months of life. Three basic cornerstones determine the individual features of Melanie Klein's theoretical framework—first, the existence of innate sexual knowledge; second, the dominant role ascribed to a primary death instinct; and third, the importance attributed to the processes of introjection and projection. From the outset, she suggests, the infant's mental life is dominated by conflict between libidinal and aggressive tendencies. In the earliest months these tendencies are related to part objects, whose significance is determined by the nature of the impulses related to them. There are, in short, good and bad part objects, related respectively to loving and aggressive impulses. Owing to the complicated interplay between processes of

[1] First published in *Affective Disorders*, edited by Phyllis Greenacre. New York: International Universities Press, 1953.

introjection and projection, these part objects are experienced both as external and as internal. Owing to the unconscious knowledge concerning the sexual relationship between the parents, this complicated interplay between processes of introjection and projection leads very soon to definite fantasies with an oedipal content. These early introjections, derived primarily from the mother's breast, but soon including the father's penis, are regarded by Melanie Klein as dynamically similar to, if not actually identical with, the definitive superego. In short, Melanie Klein pushes back the decisive conflicts regarding the oedipal conflict and superego formation to a much earlier period than is generally accepted.

A vitally important aim of all this conflict and fantasy formation is, in her opinion, the decisive and stable introjection of a predominantly good object. The earliest defences, in which good and bad part objects are separated by alternating and variable processes of introjection and projection, gradually change in important respects. In the first place, as the infant's grasp of reality develops, the part object becomes a whole object. Concurrently, and also largely dependent on reality sense, comes the realization that these good and bad objects are not really separate, but one and the same. This then brings about recognition that the love and hate which have hitherto been directed towards good and bad objects respectively are in fact directed towards the same object. The infant, that is to say, is faced with the awareness of his own aggressive destructive fantasies towards his own loved objects. This recognition then leads to fear lest his hatred and aggression prove stronger than his love, which Melanie Klein calls 'depressive fear' and, about the decisive period of weaning, to his self-reproach and depression concerning the loss of a good object, the breast, which he attributes primarily to his own destructive impulses.

This very briefly summarizes Melanie Klein's theory of the background and development of the depressive position—a subject which will be amplified later. At this point I wish to consider, first, how far the concept of the 'depressive position' is dependent on the other premises and hypotheses discussed briefly, and second, whether the various criticisms which have been or can be made in respect of her work necessarily invalidate the concept.

With respect to the first point, Melanie Klein herself would, I think, maintain that the 'depressive position' represents an integral part of her theoretical framework, and that it cannot be considered out of its context. In her view, the significance of the attainment, and the precariousness, of the good relationship with a whole good object, whether external or internal, depends on the earlier struggle, which she considers the basis of paranoid and schizophrenic reactions, with terrifying and aggressive, sadistic and masochistic fantasies concerning the relationship between the parents, the inside of the mother's body, and most important of all the infant's own internal situation resulting from wholesale introjective processes. Finally, Melanie Klein's concept of the 'depressive position' is an integral link in her developmental scheme which postulates paranoid and schizoid mechanisms at the earliest level, progressing, as whole object relations develop, to depressive fears and the depressive position, and followed by the development of important defences against the depressive position, of which the most important are the manic defence and the various processes of reparation.

After carefully examining and criticizing her theories, however, I do not feel her work to be so closely knit and interdependent that we must either accept or reject it *in toto*. With regard to the 'depressive position' in particular, I have never felt that the concept of secure object relations as gradually emerging from a struggle with conflicting feelings of love and hate, and as gradually involving recognition of the identity of the loved and hated object, necessarily rests on Melanie Klein's reconstruction of violent sadistic fantasies specifically related to the oedipal situation; nor do I feel that the dynamic concept of fear of, and reaction to, threatened loss of a good object necessarily implies acceptance of her specific views with regard to the relationship of these early introjections to definitive super-ego formation.

Since the focus of this chapter is the depressive position, we need not spend much time on Melanie Klein's general theories, important though this would be in a general discussion of her work. I will, however, state my own point of view and will also briefly consider some of the more important criticisms of her work. In the first place, the death instinct is defined and elaborated by Melanie Klein as an active destructive force originally directed against the self. This does not seem a conception in keeping with Freud's formulation, which is itself controversial. On this conception of the death instinct, at best questionable, Melanie Klein has constructed some of her most important formulations—in particular, her conception of anxiety. Other important formulations, although she would base them on the death instinct, appear equally valid on the premise of aggressive impulses. They do not, that is to say, necessarily rest on the acceptance of her hypothesis that aggression is originally directed towards the self rather than the outside world.

With regard to Melanie Klein's other basic theories—her views of early oedipal fantasies, her conception of the importance of introjective and projective processes in the mastery of the basic conflicts between love and hate, and her hypothesis as to the early development of the superego—I feel that, in spite of her boldness in approaching the mental life of the young infant, Melanie Klein's theoretical reconstructions have been marred by too faithful adherence to certain classical analytic hypotheses. To mention only a few: superego formation in the classical view occurs in relation to the Oedipus complex. In her analytic work Melanie Klein finds evidence to suggest the presence of superego-like introjections preceding the genital Oedipus complex. Two possibilities are open: first, that the precursors of the superego antedate the Oedipus complex; second, that the Oedipus complex antedates the genital level. It is the latter alternative Melanie Klein chooses. Her clinical evidence for this, although clearly illustrating the importance of oedipal fantasies with a predominantly oral or anal colouring, does not necessarily imply that these pregenital oedipal fantasies must have actually occurred at the time of oral primacy. Here her time-table is coloured by another hypothesis, namely Abraham's classification of the psychoses in terms of definite libidinal levels (1924). Although certain postulates of her work depend on her abandonment of Abraham's concept of a pre-ambivalent oral phase, Melanie Klein accepts the hypothesis that schizophrenia and paranoia antedate depression, mania and the obsessional neurosis. She produces much evidence to confirm the archaic qualities of these psychotic mechanisms. This leads her to the conclusion that the fantasies related to these processes must occur in the early months of life. In other words, Melanie Klein has entered the field with certain definite analytic preconceptions concerning the psychoses, the Oedipus complex, and superego formation; these premises have then been applied with some rigidity to her clinical findings. In particular, this attitude has played an important part in Melanie Klein's conception of unconscious knowledge and of early oedipal fantasies. Most of my remarks here are in substantial agreement with points raised by Robert Waelder in 1937.

Edward Bibring, in a more recent critical paper (1947), discusses the premises on which her reconstruction is based and shows quite convincingly the weakness of her theoretical framework. The most important premises, in his opinion, are her conception of innate unconscious knowledge and her conception of activation, which I have not discussed as it seems to me peripheral to the present discussion. Bibring concludes that

> if our criticism is valid, all those parts of the developmental reconstruction which are based on these two conceptions are bound to fall with their removal, that is, the whole structure of the early oedipal fantasies and conflicts compressed into the first six to twelve months of life (1947, p. 90 f.).

Although I substantially agree with Edward Bibring's criticism in this respect, it is the specific oedipal content of Melanie Klein's reconstruction which seems to me doubtful and unscientific, if for no other reason than that the detailed complexity she postulates seems impracticable and unbiological. I do not, however, feel that this criticism necessarily invalidates the dynamics of the mental processes Melanie Klein postulates, nor does it undermine her premises regarding the importance of the aggressive instincts from the beginning of life.

In his detailed criticism of Melanie Klein's views, Edward Glover (1945) refers to many of the questions I have raised. He amplifies and illustrates the weaknesses inherent in Melanie Klein's orientation towards the aggressive instincts; his criticism of Melanie Klein's definition of fantasy resembles in many ways Bibring's criticism of the concept of innate knowledge, and seems closely related. He also criticizes Melanie Klein's application of the concepts of fixation and regression. Although he attacks the concept of the 'depressive position' as a 'closed system'—a dubious criticism—his more important criticisms, like those of

Edward Bibring and Robert Waelder, are concerned with Melanie Klein's reconstruction of the early months of life in terms of the early spontaneous appearance of oedipal fantasies, and with the predominant role played in the structure of these fantasies by the aggressive or death instinct which she hypothesizes.

While I accept these criticisms regarding the theoretical weakness of Melanie Klein's reconstruction of the early months of life, particularly in respect of oedipal fantasies, this criticism does not necessarily undermine her conception of the 'depressive position'. Let us turn to the main topic in order to discuss in more detail Melanie Klein's views about the dynamics of mourning and the depressive states. Up to now, I have approached the concept of the 'depressive position' on the basis of her reconstructions of the growth of object relations. Now I should like to approach the topic from a more orthodox point of view and to compare her views with those of other workers. In this connection I first wish to consider two subtopics concerning which there are persistent theoretical difficulties relevant to the dynamic structure of depression. The first involves the concept of narcissism; the second relates to the process and timing of superego formation.

With respect to narcissism, it is peculiarly difficult to discuss Melanie Klein's views adequately. The reason for this is simple: Melanie Klein has practically discarded the word 'narcissism' from her vocabulary. In the few references to narcissism in the indexes of her two books, almost all are concerned with discussion or quotation of other people's work. At no point does she compare with classical theories concerning narcissistic libido her views of the relationship of libidinal development to ego and object cathexis. Although, for example, she refers briefly to Sándor Radó's paper on 'The Problem of Melancholia' (1928), she does not amplify the points of similarity and difference in this particular concept. This is a serious omission on her part—all the more important, because it seems to me that on this question her work is too significant and important not to be shown its relationship to more orthodox views. Melanie Klein has, of course, replaced the concept of narcissism by her emphasis on the importance of internal object relations. In place of the picture of the infant as an organism dominated by his need for love and security, as a primary positive need, she puts forward the concept of an infant struggling from the outset with the conflict between his loving, positive feelings, related to situations of satisfaction and fulfilment, and his aggressive, destructive feelings aroused by frustration, a significant amount of which she considers inevitable in the best feeding situation. Where most analysts would ascribe excessive need of love and reassurance (i.e. narcissistic needs) to feelings of helplessness and inadequacy, Melanie Klein would suggest that the pathogenicity of such feelings is related to the feelings of rage. These feelings, which occur at a time when the infant, it is generally agreed, cannot clearly distinguish between self and the outside world, are felt to be destructive not only to the object but to the self, or its contents, as well.

Owing to Melanie Klein's neglect of the work of other analysts on the subject of narcissism and the predisposition to depression, it is in fact difficult to assess how far her work on this particular subject represents a real departure from accepted views. If we leave aside discussion of the classical papers by Freud (1914, 1917) and Abraham (1924), we still find Sándor Radó (1928), in particular, stressing the intense ambivalence characteristic of the narcissistic struggle in the future melancholic. Georg Gerö makes very clear his recognition of this factor when he says:

> [The child's] libidinal desires are mixed with aggressive tendencies, the reactions to disappointments. His longing to be loved is too immoderate, too narcissistic; therefore it cannot be gratified. But disappointments activate his equally immoderate aggression which then must be warded off by the ego. The aggression is turned towards the self, towards the introjected object in the ego (1936, p. 458).

In spite of her insistence on the essential orthodoxy of her views in respect of the most controversial part of her work, Melanie Klein apparently does not recognize much basic similarity between contemporary important work by other workers and other parts of her work, particularly with regard to the predisposition to depression. The reason for this failure appears to me to lie in her apparently having abandoned the concept of narcissism, replacing it by emphasis on the processes of introjection and projection and on the aggressive instinct. This gives rise to real difficulties of communication, prevents mutual correlation of theoretical orientation, and inevitably exaggerates what may be at least in part *verbal* differences. My criticism here is not for the moment directed towards what I understand to be the meaning of Melanie Klein's viewpoint, but towards her failure to express her contribution in terms of its relationship to more orthodox concepts. It is not, that is to say, the fact that she has attempted to dissect and analyse the meaning of narcissism to which I object, but the fact that she has not made it clear either that this is what she is doing, or that she knows she is doing it.

Although many analysts recognize the importance of ambivalence in narcissistic needs, it seems to me that this recognition is sometimes verbal only, and that there is still a tendency to relate narcissism to a simple apparently unambivalent passive need, without due consideration of the possible relationship between this excessive need and unconscious aggressive tendencies. Bertram D. Lewin (1950), although he has elsewhere acknowledged this relationship, lays great stress in his book on what appear to be mainly positive satisfying experiences in the early months of life, with relatively little reference to the part played by conflict and ambivalence as present from the outset. Melanie Klein, on the other hand, in abandoning the concept of narcissism has gone to the other extreme. To her, the infant's idyllic experiences appear to be few and far between, and one gets the impression of an infantile mental life dominated by aggressive fantasies and the anxious or depressive reaction to them. Nevertheless, in putting forward the hypothesis that conflict predominates in mental life from the outset, she has made a very important contribution.

The second point I wish to discuss concerns the origin of the superego. Let us again set aside classical papers on this subject, since the original conception of the superego (i.e. as the heir to the genital Oedipus complex) is still accepted by most psychoanalysts. Related problems, however, have been discussed, particularly in England, not only by Melanie Klein and her followers, but also by Ernest Jones, who in his paper on 'The Origin and Structure of the Super-Ego' makes the following statement:

When, however, we leave these valuable broad generalizations and come to a closer study of some of the problems involved, a considerable number of awkward questions present themselves . . . ; there is every reason to think that the concept of the super-ego is a nodal point where we may expect all the obscure problems of the Oedipus complex and narcissism on the one hand, and hate and sadism on the other, to meet (1926, p. 188).

The problem, to put it briefly, is essentially this: how do we reconcile the hypothesis that the superego is derived from the genital Oedipus complex with the pregenital characteristics of the 'depressive superego'? Can we account for these characteristics as regressive phenomena ascribable to the pregenital fixations we know to be present in these individuals? Or can we assume that the failure to master pregenital situations has so affected superego formation from the outset that, even in relative health, the 'depressive superego' is characterized by harsh pregenital features which render the individual particularly vulnerable to any event which by lowering self-esteem will push the pathological superego into melancholic self-reproach? Finally, is it not possible that in depressive illness regression takes place to the now generally accepted precursors of the definitive superego which represent the introjection and identifications of the pregenital period?

The problem before us here, too, is the explanation not only of the oral, pregenital nature of the 'depressive superego', but also of the generally recognized oral features of the oedipal situation itself found in the analysis of these patients. It is generally agreed—the emphasis given this subject in all discussions of the subject points to a consensus of opinion—that the question of superego formation is a crucial point in this problem.

I should like at this point to recapitulate Melanie Klein's views on the matter. She gives, briefly, the following answers: the archaic pregenital nature of the superego in these patients points to the possibility that the definitive superego has antecedents, structurally comparable, which are formed at pregenital levels. In melancholic individuals, because of failure to master the conflicts of this period, superego structure retains these archaic characteristics which reappear in the regression of melancholic illness. The presence of oedipal fantasies of a predominantly oral nature she would explain not as a regressive phenomenon attributable to the disease process, but as illustrating the presence in the early months of life of oedipal fantasies of a predominantly oral and sadistic nature.

In discussing the same basic problem, Edith Jacobson comes to a different conclusion. In her opinion

> the super-ego may be called a compound of Oedipus-strivings and prohibitions as well as a compromise with regard to the infantile narcissistic desires: It denies the child the desired parental omnipotence, yet sets up the god image within the ego. . . . This is accomplished by regressive reanimation of the originally omnipotent parental images . . . (1946, p. 134).

In other words, the archaic nature of the 'depressive superego' does not necessarily point to pregenital superego functions. It is rather attributable to regressive processes, precipitated by disappointment at the oedipal level, which reanimate the introjections of an earlier period. It is relevant to note here Edith Jacobson's assumption that early pregenital parental introjections, however activated, play a decisive part in superego formation. It is also worth noting that she too raises the possibility of premature superego formation in the future depressive.

To Edith Jacobson, an oedipal situation complicated by severe disappointment in both parents may, in an individual of depressive predisposition, be decisive both for superego formation and for the probability of future depressive illness. Melanie Klein would, I think, agree in accepting the importance of disappointment in the parents at this critical period: she would, however, be concerned to elucidate the *significance* to the child of this disappointment in the light of its own fantasies and fears. Edith Jacobson, for example, lays great stress on the pathogenic significance of devalued, useless parents—as contrasted with that of powerful parents—whether for good or evil. She postulates an identification with these devalued, useless parents which leads to diminution of the ego and the sense of worthlessness so characterististic of the depressive. She would, however, regard the precipitating event in this pathogenic chain of events as emanating from some real failure on the part of the parents. Melanie Klein, on the other hand, while accepting the real disappointment, would relate its pathogenic effect to the mental state of the child at the time of the disappointment in the specific sense that she would attribute the child's depressive reaction to its feeling of guilt and responsibility for the parents' failure. The devalued parents, which both Edith Jacobson and Melanie Klein agree to be introjected into the ego, would, according to Melanie Klein's point of view, represent the damaged or destroyed parents, or combined parental figure; the child, in short, would attribute the parental disappointment to its own aggression and hostility.

In considering these problems concerning the structure of melancholia and its relation to the nature of narcissism and to early superego formation, we have touched on some of the more important work on the subject and compared certain aspects of Melanie Klein's views with those of other workers. So far, however, attention has been directed mainly to the structure and meaning of pathological depression and to the nature of the problem Melanie Klein is attempting to solve. I have not as yet discussed in any detail the most controversial aspect of Melanie Klein's views on depression, namely her concept of the 'depressive position' as a normal phenomenon in infantile life. To do this, let us once more return to the question of mourning and melancholia. In her work on this subject Melanie Klein has made two significant suggestions. In the first place she has suggested that the differences between mourning and melancholia, although decisive for the mental health of the individual, are not so great as has sometimes been averred. In her extremely interesting description of the experience of a normal mourner she illustrates particularly by dream analysis how, in a brief, modified form (which is eventually overcome by healthy defences and reparative processes), the mental state of the mourner is comparable in every respect with that of the melancholic. There is, unconsciously, definite evidence of self-reproachful processes, guilt with regard to the death of the lost love object, devaluation of the self. There is, too, a sense of triumph with subsequent guilt which is clearly related to aggressive fantasies. Gradually, however, the normal mourner is able to set up within himself a predominantly positive introjection of the lost love object, and when this is accomplished the work of mourning is more or less complete. Melanie Klein also gives a good deal of material illustrating how the real external loss revives or reactivates in the individual his earlier struggles of a similar nature, most of which appeared referable to the earliest relation with the mother. In the normal mourner, that is to say, the real object loss revives this decisive previous struggle. In individuals who have made an early satisfactory solution with subsequent good object relationships, mourning is successfully accomplished. In others, where this early struggle resulted in comparative failure and difficulties in accomplishing good object relationships, the reaction to loss will approach more or less closely a clinical depression.

In speaking of Melanie Klein's formulations regarding pathological conditions (particularly the more severe depressive illnesses in which the part played by real object loss is obscure and unrecognized) one must express considerable reserve. Her adult patients, for the most part, appear to be severe neurotics, personality problems, and examples of typical neurotic depression. In my opinion the differences between these cases and the more severe patients seen in hospitals are neither straightforward nor predominantly quantitative. Melanie Klein underestimates the importance both of constitutional factors and of the complexity of the process of maturation. My attitude seems to be in accord with Edward Bibring's emphasis on the part played by complicating factors in determining the different clinical manifestations of depression. Bibring, however, has also emphasized the fundamental unity of the basic feelings of depression (see 1947, pp. 13–48). He showed that in spite of the wide range between mild sadness, mourning and feeling of disinterest—many of which are within the scope of normal experience—and the various pathological conditions in which depression is a presenting symptom, there is a basic unity of the depressive process. With this point of view Melanie Klein would be in agreement, although her conception of the dynamics of these basic feelings differs from his in important respects.

This unitary conception of depression, however, makes it essential that we be very clear as to Melanie Klein's meaning when she postulates the existence of depressive tendencies as a normal phenomenon of infantile life. It is, in short, particularly important to ascertain whether, in talking of the 'infantile depressive position', she is comparing the infant with the adult melancholic or with the normal mourner. Some of the objections to her conception arise from a misunderstanding of this crucial point. Granted that there are accepted resemblances between mourning and melancholia, the crucial differences between them must always be borne in mind. Mourning, however painful, is—no matter how much its dynamic unconscious structure resembles that of pathogenic illness—a normal human experience which few of us escape. No one who has either undergone this experience with psychological insight into his own mental state, or who has had an opportunity of analysing someone immediately after bereavement, could fail to confirm much that Melanie Klein says about the ambivalent reactions related to the introjection of the lost love object, and, most important from our point of view, about the revival of primitive feelings of conflict and dependence on the mother. Melanie Klein, in postulating the conception of an early 'depressive position' as crucial, not only in relation to the reaction to real object loss, but for the development of good object relations throughout life, is referring to the manner in which the weaning process constitutes a real object loss. She is offering the hypothesis that the attainment of a predominantly positive object relationship prior to this first object loss is crucial for future development. That is to say, the infant must, during the weaning process, come to terms with a real object loss (i.e. the loss of the breast or its substitute). This is the basis for the concept of a 'depressive position'. Now this loss, like the real losses of later life, is an inevitable event in human development and one which, it is generally accepted, is of great emotional significance for the child. What determines its successful or unsuccessful outcome? And what is the significance of this conflict for future mental health, with particular reference to depression? It is in the answers to these questions that the significance of Melanie Klein's approach becomes clear. Melanie Klein suggests that—just as with the adult mourner—it is the successful introjection of a predominantly good object which is the goal. Where, however, the relatively greater strength of the aggressive impulses prevents this occurrence the introjected good object is felt to be lost, and is, typically, replaced by the hostile damaged or destroyed objects which so closely resemble the devalued parents described by Edith Jacobson. Between these two extremes occur the infinite variations in object relationship which are so familiar.

Not only psychoanalysts, but anthropologists, psychologists and pediatricians, have in recent years stressed with increasing vigour the importance of the early mother–child relationship for the successful development of the human infant. There are, of course, differences of opinion as to how far either success on the one hand, or failure on the other, plays a decisive role in the later crucial emotional struggles of childhood. In spite of the real difficulties of proving in our analytic work how far our reconstructions of preverbal mental life are valid, I think we would all agree as to the importance of the experiences of these early months in providing or not providing a foundation of security and positive feeling as the basis for future object relationships. Most of the work on this subject has stressed the infant's basic need—indeed inherent right—to the security which appears to be such a basic requirement. That undue frustration predisposes to a variety of pathological developments is also generally accepted.

René Spitz (1946), in his interesting and important contributions on the psychopathology of infancy, has clearly demonstrated the overt depressive states precipitated in infants forcibly separated from their mothers during the second six months of life. In these cases, to the inevitable struggle over the loss of the breast was added the concurrent loss of the mother as a whole—a situation differing decisively from that of the normal infant, where, as Melanie Klein points out, 'The whole situation and the defences of the baby, who obtains reassurance over and over again in the love of the mother, differ greatly from those in the adult melancholic' (1935, p. 307). The fact that loss of the mother during this decisive period produces actual clinical depression seems to me evidence in favour of the depressive vulnerability of the infant at this point. Other observers, too, have noted the decisive change in the baby's relationship to its mother at or about six months, and they agree as to the special vulnerability of the baby to separation from its mother at the time when he comes to know her as a whole person.

In his paper Edward Bibring (1947) suggests that the source or anlage of depressive symptoms may be sought in the feelings of helplessness of the infant in the face of frustration. It is possible that he, too, might be inclined to agree that the critical period for this experience is related to the emergence of a whole object relationship where the need and desire are first related to a specific individual, the mother. The decisive problem for us, however, is to decide how far this recognized dependence of the infant on security and gratification implies that reactions of helplessness and rage constitute a response to a specific traumatic experience of frustration and rejection on the part of the mother. This is implicit in most orthodox opinions. The alternative proposed by Melanie Klein is that the degree of depressive anxiety aroused by greater or less external frustration will depend not only on the environmental situation but on the infant's anxieties regarding his own aggressive tendencies. Let us, for the sake of simplification, accept for the moment the proposition that, at or about the time of weaning, the infant has developed a real enough object relationship with its mother to feel helpless, frightened or depressed at her threatened or actual loss. Should we explain this reaction as a simple maturational phenomenon, a reaction which must inevitably occur when the infant comes to know his mother and his own dependence on her for gratification? Or should we, on the other hand, believe that, in addition to these maturational processes, there has already been a gradual psychological development from part to whole object relationship and that during this period, characterized by confusion between outer and inner worlds and conflicts between love and hate, introjective and projective processes have played an important part? In other words, how far should we agree with Melanie Klein that the infant during the early sucking period believes or fears that the absent breast is gone because it is inside him?

We find ourselves here in the realm of reconstruction, since up to the present no scientific proof has been possible. From observations of young infants there has been some suggestive evidence. Most of our information, however, is derived—as I think it must be—from our analytic work. To me, and to many British-trained analysts who have been stimulated by Melanie Klein's work but who have not joined her followers, her conception of the growth of object relationships in an ambivalent setting is her most valuable contribution. There is much clinical material compatible with the concept that the struggle between love and hate leads to depressive fears lest the hating impulses prove the stronger. One common analytic example of this type of material is concerned with the struggle to maintain a good object relationship in the transference situation in spite of negative feelings often aroused by the analyst's absence or lateness. Most typical of all, perhaps, are feelings aroused in connection with the temporary breaks during vacation periods. The importance of this material lies not in its rarity but in its ubiquity. The intensity of these reactions varies from a true, though temporary, depression to feelings of mild anxiety where the depressive content reveals itself only in dreams. The decisive factor in determining the quality and pathogenicity of these reactions is clearly related to the degree to which the individual is capable of tolerating his own recognition of ambivalence without feeling over-anxious lest his hate prove stronger than his love. In more disturbed patients, particularly in those with underlying, often unconscious depressive features, the inability to tolerate this conflict is repeatedly demonstrated by, for example, excessively positive feelings expressed during analytic sessions, with a tendency to react to the analyst's absence even over weekends with fears lest he is or is about to be maimed or destroyed. That this material is related to early feeding situations has been strongly suggested in certain cases, both by the oral content of the material and by a known history of early feeding problems with a lifelong ambivalence of object relationships.

How far can we assume that these ambivalent reactions to frustration and loss in either child or adult patients must be regarded as partial or complete repetitions of earlier reactions? A similar and crucial scientific question also remains as to how far we are justified in assuming that material which appears to be deepest, both in difficulty of access and in its archaic structure, is necessarily earliest from the developmental point of view. It is certain that Melanie Klein has pushed both these premises to their utmost limits and beyond the point where any satisfactory method of validation has yet been discovered. I wish to stress once more that I do not believe that either Melanie Klein's theoretical framework, or her specific reconstructions regarding the content of infantile fantasies, constitutes her most significant contribution to analytic thought. Her formulations are attempts to verbalize material which is fundamentally preverbal in nature —an attempt which is coloured by her efforts to couch her formulations within the framework of more or less orthodox analytic hypotheses.

A possible explanation is that vague and often diffuse bodily and emotional experiences related to the parents, which may in the early months of life enter into and colour the later oedipal situation in important respects, are treated as if these later conflicts had already been present at the earlier period. This happens because during analysis, and probably particularly during the analysis of children at or about the crucial oedipal period, the material presents itself as if the nursing infant had experienced the fantasies expressed so clearly by the four- or five-year-old. That is to say, while the material is true, it is not necessarily correct in timing, owing to the retrospective oedipal interpretation of earlier experiences.

As I see it, the decisive question concerns the nature and origin of mental conflict in the human infant. At first glance Melanie Klein's conception of the aggressive instincts raises objections from a biological and commonsense point of view. The whole science of psychoanalysis, however, derives from what might be called the unbiological and uncommonsensical nature of the human being. It seems to me a hypothesis worth full examination—namely, that the combination of excessive helplessness with the infant's capacity for more or less distinct awareness of this situation long before the development of any effective mode of reaction or defence—may well result in the early appearance, not only of aggressive impulses, which are well recognized, but also of psychological attempts to explain experience in the light of these conflicting emotions, i.e. fantasies, or perhaps better the preverbal precursors of fantasies. Moreover, we have much analytic experience to suggest that along with these feelings of helplessness there exist important and significant feelings of omnipotence, which refer not only to the positive power to fantasy the wished-for breast, for example, but also negative convictions that the absence itself has been brought about by an omnipotent destructive impulse.

In considering Melanie Klein's views I have tried to separate her theoretical framework, which is often obscure and in many respects controversial, from what appear to me the more significant aspects of her approach to the problem of depression in relation to the development of object relations and early mental conflict. Although her point of view raises a number of vitally important issues—in particular, the nature of narcissism, the role of the aggressive instincts, and the development of the superego—much of her work need not necessarily imply an important departure from orthodox analytic views. Finally, with regard to the concept of the 'depressive position' I feel that more than anything else the term is unfortunate, since it seems to imply more far-reaching implications of infantile psychosis than is in fact the case. As suggested, there seems to be a good deal of work to substantiate her conception that the achievement of a whole object relationship is accompanied by anxiety and a definite and specific vulnerability to depression in the event of object loss. In this sense, then, the concept of the 'depressive position'—under some more suitable name (I would suggest the term 'depressive vulnerability')—may prove a concept of considerable importance in our growing knowledge of the development of object relations.

To sum up: in this chapter Melanie Klein's concept of the 'depressive position' is approached from two points of view. In the first place her general theoretical orientation is considered with special reference to the development of the 'depressive position', with subsequent consideration of how far this concept is separable from the whole context of her theories and whether or not criticism directed against these theories necessarily invalidates the 'depressive position'. In the second place, important views on the subject of depression are discussed in comparison with Melanie Klein's. In doing this, I have tried to relate the concept of the 'depressive position' to normal mourning. For reasons of brevity many important aspects of her work—in particular, her conception of mania and of the processes of reparation—have been omitted.

It may seem that by pruning Melanie Klein's work I have left relatively little that is objectionable. But since, after all, other workers—Radó, Gerö, Jacobson, to mention only a few—have also stressed the significance of ambivalent struggles in early childhood in relation to depression, little seems left that is important or individual. My wish has been to evaluate the scientific validity of Melanie Klein's views in the light of our present state of knowledge. It is always essential in any science, but perhaps particularly in our own, to remember to distinguish between that which we believe to be true and which, as far our as powers of validation go, we feel proved to be true, and that which offers suggestive and fruitful hypotheses which may be true but which must so far be considered unproved. Melanie Klein's views, although they offer dynamic and stimulating hypotheses, belong to the latter category. It is safe to say that few who have worked with her have failed to be impressed by her immediacy of insight into the deeper levels of the unconscious mind. Her interpretations of the dreams, fantasies and the associations of numerous patients have resulted in a considerable body of evidence regarding the existence and importance of many of the conflicts she hypothesizes. Nevertheless there is a considerable step between recognizing and interpreting specific unconscious material, and hypothesizing a theoretical reconstruction with far-reaching implications. Melanie Klein's theoretical framework is based not only on her clinical findings but on her specific premises regarding the basic instincts and archaic mental processes. In so far, therefore, as these premises are not regarded as proved, her theoretical framework cannot be considered to rest on a sound basis. It would, however, be unfortunate for the development of psychoanalysis if Melanie Klein's controversial theoretical approach, and occasional verbal obscurity, should lead us to forget the importance and significance of her dynamic approach to the problems of early infantile development.

6

ON THE INCAPACITY TO BEAR DEPRESSION[1]

(1965)

As I suggested in Chapter 3, manifest anxiety, however painful or temporarily disabling, should not be evaluated exclusively in the light of its pathological implications. In development, tolerance and mastery should rather be understood as essential both to the developmental process and to the maintenance of sustained mental health. In that earlier chapter I concluded that the distinction between anxiety as a manifestation of something which has not been tolerated resulting in psychic disaster, and anxiety as the purposive response to a threatened danger which has not yet taken place, throws considerable light on many problems. At that time, however, I did not discuss the closely related problems of the tolerance of guilt and depression.

This bears indirectly on the dual goal of the present chapter. On the one hand, I hope to confirm and to amplify the adaptive value of certain manifestations of psychic distress which is experienced and mastered in an appropriate developmental context. On the other, my developmental approach here emphasizes the role of certain basic affects.[2]

By way of introduction, the gradually emerging thesis underlying my more recent contributions treating these matters may here be appropriately summarized. Expansions of the developmental hypothesis increasingly touch on psychoanalytic ego psychology. In the first place, the quality of the dyadic object relations that dominate the pre-oedipal period is reflected throughout life in certain basic attributes of definitive character

[1] First published, under the title 'Depression and the Incapacity to Bear It', in *Drives, Affects, Behavior*, Volume 2, edited by Max Schur. New York: International Universities Press, 1965.

[2] During the years since 1949 I have approached such problems from somewhat different angles in a number of papers (see Chapters 4, 5, 10 and 11).

structure and function. In the second place, the developmental process must be understood as a lifelong phenomenon. Though the achievements and failures of early childhood have certain permanent after-effects, the maturational challenges and regressive dangers of later critical periods impose repeated problems. The healthy or pathological solutions achieved earlier influence the psychological resources available to the individual at each successive developmental phase. The demand that the individual master crucial psychological conflicts is not limited to the early years of childhood.

Adolescence, for example, is a time when partial solutions, adequate during the latency period, are undermined by the onset of sexual maturity. This explains the widely recognized pathology of this period of life. Yet the reopening of a previously closed book offers the individual a new opportunity to reach a higher level of emotional maturity. Similar considerations apply to later developmental periods. In early maturity, with the demand to choose a career and select a life partner, unresolved early conflicts often lead to manifest symptom formation. Parenthood revives in both sexes infantile, dependent wishes coincident with the added responsibilities and increased complexity of family life. The involutional period and its pathology are too well known to require emphasis. Retirement, old age and imminent death are also periods of life for which psychoanalysis has specified comprehensive developmental psychology.

Our developmental hypothesis assumes a psychic apparatus capable of progessive and regressive responses to both external and internal challenge and change. The two responses are not mutually exclusive; they may, in fact, be inextricably combined. Moreover, just as anxiety has healthy as well as pathological attributes, so regression—as Ernst Kris (1950) and others have demonstrated—is not exclusively pathological. We may, in fact, consider regression an essential concomitant of learning, of the creative process and of genuine insight in the course of clinical psychoanalysis. Regression characterized by symptom formation may, in potentially healthy individuals, represent a temporary reverse preceding conflict solution and increased emotional maturity. Understanding that symptoms and pathological ego defences may be attempts to resolve problems can be illuminating as regards both classical symptom formation in the neuroses, and the more severe disturbances seen in serious character disorders and overt psychoses. The adaptive hypothesis, within this context, applies not only to external, interpersonal responses, but also to the intrapsychic mechanisms available at each developmental level. External adjustment does not always imply internal stability or mature achievement. Nor is psychopathology to be measured in terms of immediate symptomatology or distress. Both should rather be evaluated within the framework of their developmental implications.

Such an evaluation was implicit in Chapter 3. I had noted in the clinical observation of many hundreds of neurotic soldiers the adaptive and prophylactic value of previously tolerated overt anxiety. Broadly based empirical observations thus led to theoretical deductions, many of which have since been confirmed or amplified by other contributors. Erik Erikson (1950) considers anxiety and its mastery indispensable for the achievement and maintenance of emotional maturity.

Phyllis Greenacre (1941) differentiates between those early factors that lead to a basic, relatively unalterable predisposition to anxiety and the later infantile neurosis that may be interpreted as the response to signal anxiety. The first concerns factors limiting the capacity to bear anxiety. The second concerns areas in which intrapsychic defences have been established. Limitations determined by the earlier developmental failure, however, influence the degree to which persons predisposed to great anxiety can respond successfully to traditional psychoanalytic technique. Other recent discussions concerning clinical criteria have emphasized the indispensability of the ability to tolerate anxiety for the development and resolution of an analysable transference neurosis. As I stated in Chapter 3, the capacity to recognize and tolerate the existence of an internal, unconsciously determined danger situation is very closely linked with the problem of psychological insight. In the analysis of neurotic patients, this capacity of achieving and tolerating the anxiety associated with insight is of decisive importance.

Theoretical contributions closely related to both the earlier and the current discussion have been presented in a series of papers by Max Schur (1953, 1955). These have particularly enriched and expanded—from the point of view of ego psychology—questions previously raised in a somewhat different context. Contained anxiety, as Schur defines it, seems essentially synonymous with a degree of secondary anxiety that does not exceed individual capacity to bear it. As anxiety mounts, we may discern the emergence of more primitive manifestations, defined in terms of Freud's concept of primary anxiety (1926). Max Schur (1953) emphasizes two major qualities of ego regression with respect to anxiety: first, the re-emergence of primary-process discharge at the expense of secondary-process ideation; and second, a related, increasingly primitive evaluation of danger as the ego regresses. Somatization, though precipitated by intrapsychic events, utilizes physical channels as a means of discharge. The regressive evaluation, if it proceeds unchecked, may result in an impairment of reality testing and may eventually reach psychotic proportions. As self-object differentiation is impaired, the capacity to recognize and respond to signal anxiety disappears. Ego defences against internal danger no longer adequately explain either the quality of affective distress or the symptoms experienced in such regressive states. Freud concluded: 'I can see no objection to there being a twofold origin of anxiety—one as a direct consequence of the traumatic moment and the other as a signal threatening a repetition of such a moment' (1933, p. 94 f.). An analogy is here implicit between the comparable differentiation between the primary form (repression) and the secondary form (identification) of narcissism. Generally speaking, the former precedes self-object differentiation and the distinction between external and internal reality. So, too, the traumatic situation (primary anxiety) has its roots in the earliest period of neonatal life. Signal anxiety, by contrast, is contingent on considerable ego development. In this sense, the term 'secondary anxiety' has much to recommend it.

The capacity to tolerate and master the secondary anxiety depends on definitive attributes of the mature psychic apparatus. Persons whose capacity is limited by relative developmental failure and those whose disposition to anxiety is excessive respond by the regressive changes Schur described. The wide variety of both somatic and psychic symptoms, the shifting of emphasis from one to the other, and the different responses to therapeutic intervention all indicate the complexity of psychic events that may intervene between Freud's sharply differentiated primary and secondary forms of anxiety (1926). This reinforces another suggestion made earlier in Chapter 3: 'Between the type of anxiety or fear which is entirely successful in its stimulating effects and the type of anxiety which is entirely inhibiting there is a wide range of conditions which comprise the various types of clinical anxiety, and the defences against them.'

Maxwell Gitelson (1958*a*), referring to this proposed intermediate area, suggested that in addition to psychosomatic reactions, certain borderline character traits might be attributable to a similar relative developmental failure. It is pertinent to this discussion that Gitelson not only notes the adaptive value of many pathological ego distortions but also emphasizes the positive value of sustained 'object hunger' as a prophylactic against ultimate psychic disaster.

Before elaborating on the relevance of Gitelson's comments to the tolerance of depression, let us consider the nature and significance of traumatic experience as a psychic disaster. The qualitative difference between both contained secondary anxiety and anxiety in the intermediate area, and the affect experienced in a traumatic situation was emphasized in Chapter 3. In addition, the regressive after-effects of traumatic experience—depression, hypochondriasis and mild paranoid tendencies—were described as reactions to a psychic disaster. The traumatic experience, I concluded, is closely related to helplessness in a situation where the individual not only feels abandoned by all good objects, but subject to attack by all bad ones. In such states, whether internally or externally determined, the sustained 'object hunger' referred to by Gitelson is no longer present. The kind of helplessness which characterizes traumatic experience leads us to the ego-psychological approach to depression outlined by Edward Bibring (1953), who proposed that both anxiety and depression are basic ego states, which are, however, diametrically opposed in many ways. The ego, he suggests, responds to anxiety as a threat that mobilizes all available resources. In contrast, it appears to be helpless in depressive states: the threatened danger either has already materialized or is passively accepted as inevitable. The ego modification, however slight, involves loss of self-esteem associated with the sense of helplessness which is experienced as a narcissistic injury.

Understanding of the unconscious significance of prolonged depression in the post-traumatic states is much enriched by these considerations. The subjective helplessness integral to traumatic experience has obvious depressive implications. Depressive responses after the acute experience are therefore to be anticipated. In persons whose previous self-esteem has not been contingent on absence of subjective anxiety, depressive responses are, as a rule, temporary and reversible. Recollection of the traumatic experience does not in such cases involve a permanent narcissistic injury, since awareness and acceptance of potential helplessness in the face of overwhelming stress or disaster had previously been integrated into the perception of internal and external reality.

In contrast, individuals whose pre-traumatic self-esteem has depended on lack of anxiety and an underlying conviction of relative omnipotence find themselves in a much different situation. While they can no longer deny feelings of inadequacy and fear, they cannot accept and integrate the recollection of traumatic experience. Since they are neither so strong nor so brave as they had previously believed, they can no longer maintain their narcissistic ideals (Bibring, 1953). Characteristically, they are also unable to accept the proposition that strength and bravery of the order they had assumed is not realistically attainable. Underlying depression may, in such cases, be overshadowed by the litigious search for compensation so familiar in the manifest symptomatology of post-traumatic neurosis. External events and realistic injury are held responsible for the continued disability. Since the pre-traumatic self-image is not only maintained, but retrospectively enhanced, relative developmental failure precludes the acceptance of realistic limitations. This failure to achieve such acceptance is one prototype of depression and the incapacity to bear it.

My major purpose here is to introduce a developmental evaluation of depression parallel to Schur's (1953) discriminating discussion of anxiety and parallel to my own earlier discussion. However slight its overt expression may be, the experience of depression is a prerequisite for optimal maturation. Depressive affect comparable to contained anxiety occurs in response to loss, disappointment, frustration, illness, retirement, and other painful, though inevitable, experiences. As depression increases, loss of self-esteem is compounded, in predisposed individuals, by the increased severity of a regressive, sadistic superego. Finally, the perception of reality, both external and internal, may be so regressively impaired that psychosis becomes manifest. The person perceives himself as both helpless and hopeless, and the outside world as rejecting and malignant. The inability to contain or to tolerate depression leads to an outcome very similar to the end state of uncontained anxiety—thus ideas of reference, projection and delusion formation frequently bear evidence of the inability to tolerate depression. Denial, also, is a primitive defence by means of which the perception of both external and internal reality is regressively changed.

We may understand depression, of whatever degree, as a basic ego state characterized by loss of self-esteem. Despite this common feature, we must nonetheless make a clinical differentiation between depression as a reactive symptom, depressive illness as a syndrome, and depressive character structure. The first corresponds generally to contained secondary anxiety. The second is comparable to ego regression in anxiety. The third is closely related to predisposition to anxiety (see Greenacre, 1941). Depression, like anxiety, represents an ego response to internal or external events. It may lead to an adaptive progressive move toward greater psychic maturity. It also, however, frequently becomes manifest as maladaptive, regressive illness determined by earlier developmental failure. In evaluating symptomatic depression a major consideration is the degree to which immediate distress may offer an opportunity for adaptive mastery and maturation. In clinical practice the capacity of the depressed patient to seek help and subsequently to achieve a positive therapeutic alliance is of prognostic importance. Many psychotic depressives, despite verbal demands for help, are unable to achieve or to maintain any meaningful object relationships.

Whatever the precipitating cause of the depression, the quality and stability of previous object relations, the capacity to renounce an omnipotent self-image, and acceptance of the limitations of reality appear to be decisive areas. Depression in an individual whose development in these areas has been satisfactory seldom reaches psychotic proportions. Persons whose object relations have been highly ambivalent, whose self-esteem has been dependent either on successful performance or on excessive gratification, appear, on the other hand, to be highly vulnerable. Psychotic depression thus is the outcome of a failure to experience and master the depression inevitable in developmental crises.

Whether and how far therapeutic intervention may prove effective appears to be a function of both the degree of early failure and the extent of regression at the time of evaluation.

An account of a recent therapeutic contact with a patient suffering from a psychotic depressive illness may illustrate this statement. When I first saw this woman, she presented all the symptoms of a classical involutional depression. Severely depressed, retarded and self-reproachful, she exhibited marked diurnal fluctuation. She had lost faith in her religion, and she denounced herself as unable to love. At the same time, however, she expressed considerable anger towards her parents and her husband, whom she held responsible for many of her problems. She sought psychiatric help with great reluctance, having been convinced all her life that to seek help was a sign of weakness. At our first meeting her inability to form a genuine (object) relationship made it impossible to establish an effective therapeutic situation. Her symptoms, moreover, were so severe and incapacitating that to treat her as an outpatient or to confine treatment to psychotherapeutic intervention was impossible. Despite her distrust, however, she was able to achieve sufficient confidence in her therapist to accept hospitalization and the physical measures of the indicated treatment. After a relatively brief hospitalization she made a symptomatic recovery. Despite an initial attempt to take flight into health and to withdraw from therapeutic contact, she had gained enough insight to accept the advice that she should continue having some regular interviews. After several months' remission, her depression recurred. She became retarded and somewhat depressed, with the other concomitant characteristics of depressive illness. During this relapse, however, there was no recurrence of the psychotic ideation seen in her earlier decompensation. She maintained regular contact with her therapist, accepted advice, and effectively utilized certain clarifications. Hospitalization was not necessary, and the illness, though moderately disabling, followed a relatively benign course. That she had been able to maintain a positive relationship during a period of depression led, furthermore, to added personal insight and greater emotional maturity. Unlike the first depression, the second illness was essentially contained. There are still further indications that this patient had made substantial progress in respect of her capacity for positive object relations, her ability to accept limitations, and her capacity to tolerate depression without significant ego regression.

This brief history suggests the possibility of a justifiable, though limited, optimism concerning anticipated therapeutic goals for patients first seen relatively late in life. Despite earlier failures, which had determined a relatively severe ego regression, this patient was able to establish a stable therapeutic alliance. She was, moreover, able to contain a second depression and to use therapy effectively to protect her against repetition of the withdrawal, self-punishment and anger that had characterized her earlier illness. Her positive response suggests, first, the critical importance of a sustained, positive object relationship in determining the capacity to tolerate depression, and second, the continued possibility of added psychic maturation subsequent to regressive responses that may have first become manifest rather late in life.

It is probable that this patient, like many others, will need a sustained therapeutic relationship for some time. Psychotherapy involving a regressive-dependent transference, however, is neither indicated nor desirable. Though unresolved oedipal problems may have contributed to her object choice and to other problems in her immediate family situation, she had been able to function effectively with considerable satisfaction before the onset of her illness. The availability of a trusted object and her emerging capacity to accept some limited dependence appear to have increased rather than decreased her basic self-esteem. When she could come to better terms with her own internal limitations, her interest in and empathy with others significantly increased. Her illness and treatment appear to have strengthened rather than weakened her ego structure and function. In this sense her depression, despite its painful incapacitating symptomatology, represents a potential step towards greater adaptation and self-mastery.

In suggesting that this patient's ego maturation in the involutional period depended on her establishing a new and qualitatively different type of object relationship, I am approaching an area of importance to the understanding of depression. In Chapter 7 I conclude that it may prove extremely difficult to conceptualize the meaning of early object relations in terms of our present conceptual framework. It may indeed prove that psychoanalytic truth cannot be adequately expressed in abstract conceptual terms based on the individual psychic apparatus.

Many fundamental questions concerning this earliest period of psychic development still remain unanswered. Just as Max Schur's discussion (1953) of anxiety hints at complex developmental variations that may intervene between primary and secondary anxiety, a parallel approach to depression deals with psychic events in the same intermediate area. This developmental approach to both anxiety and depression highlights the effect of early object relations on basic ego functions and the tolerance of affect. While up to this point depression and anxiety have been discussed mainly in terms attributable to regressive changes within the individual psychic apparatus, since signal anxiety remains the precipitating stimulus (despite the emergence of regressive changes that modify the perception of danger) these changes may ultimately lead to a situation in which external and internal threats can no longer be clearly distinguished. Comparably, the narcissistic injury which determines the onset of depression may also lead to primitive responses impairing the perception of reality.

Contained anxiety or contained depression may not seriously hamper object relations. The regressive features already noted, however, are not all characterized by significant modifications. As the ego regresses, anxiety serves less and less effectively as the motive for intrapsychic defences—however pathological. The increased demands for external support and reassurance characteristic of severe phobic patients were noted by Helene Deutsch (1929), who emphasized such patients' need for a protective companion, often the mother or her surrogate. Approaching the subject mainly from the point of view of instinctual development, she delineated an ambivalent relationship with the mother attributable to unresolved pregenital conflicts. We know that the excessive demands expressed by severely anxious patients present grave problems for treatment and management. As regression continues, the demands tend to become highly unrealistic, which process leads to inevitable frustration. This frustration, which the patient experiences as rejection, represents a narcissistic injury that may undermine a highly vulnerable sense of self-esteem. It also increases aggression, guilt and the sense of helplessness characteristic of depressive states. Clinical practitioners know that the frantic demands of patients in states of uncontained anxiety closely resemble the agitated pressure shown by many psychotically depressed patients. In both, excessive demands for support, reassurance and attention indicate that regressive changes in the ego include increasing impairment of the capacity for stable object relations.

It is well known that many regressive states include components of both anxiety and depression. Despite the marked overt differences between the two, we must recognize the existence of an area of overlap. There is an area of psychic distress distinguished by both the sense of helplessness characteristic of depression and the desperate attempts to obtain relief, which include all the psychic and somatic features of severe anxiety. Whether this form of distress can be alleviated by appropriate therapeutic intervention depends on the degree to which object hunger is maintained. If, despite feelings of helplessness, loss of self-esteem and underlying depression, the patient maintains some genuine capacity for a sustained object relationship, he may avoid regression of psychotic proportions. In this context Ralph Greenson's (1959) suggestion that the prototype of depression occurs at a later stage of psychic development than the prototype of primary anxiety seems relevant. This does not, however, imply the incompatibility of these two basic affects, which incompatibility he appears to support.

His suggestion is compatible with the classical analytic papers which have discussed depression from the point of view of instinctual maturation. The critical period for depression appears to parallel the 'intermediate area' of anxiety. It is characterized by externally directed objective anxiety rather than by intrapsychic responses to a signal. In 'Beyond the Pleasure Principle' (1920) Freud reported on the observation of a baby, material that touches closely on the topic of this chapter. He there described the repetitive play in relation to the concept of the repetition compulsion. The same material illustrates retrospectively the function of transitional objects in the mastery of separation from known and important individuals. Over-investment in such transitional objects frequently indicates earlier developmental failure. The exploitation of real people as transitional objects has recently been discussed by Arnold Modell (1963). The object hunger refers to a related phenomenon.

Genuine mastery of separation and disappointment demands recognition of the inanimate nature of the concrete object and continued genuine investment in a real person. As a hypothesis for discussion, let us suppose that the healthy, mature individual has worked through certain crucial experiences which lead to the acceptance of both his own limitations and the limitations of reality. This enhances his capacity to tolerate, without significant ego regression, depressive affect attributable to real experiences of loss, disappointment and frustration. There is much to suggest that this developmental task is initiated between the end of the first year of life and the onset of the genital oedipal situation. The time span of many months necessary for this achievement shows that repeated experiences must be integrated. The qualitative differences between reactions approaching traumatic experience and those indicating initial active mastery based on tolerance of painful affect may be illustrated by brief descriptions of similar observations reported by the mothers of two little boys between one and two years of age.

The first illustrates acute primitive distress comparable to mixed states of anxiety and depression in adult life. This little boy's father went on a week's vacation, leaving his wife and child at home. The child, who did not talk very much, constantly repeated the word 'Daddy', and eagerly looked at pictures of his father. During most of the day he appeared to be happy and contented. Towards the end of the week, however, he began to show periods of acute distress around the time when his father usually came home from work. On one such occasion a friend of the mother's, well known to the child, came to visit her at just about this time. The little boy suddenly showed distress in which anxiety, rage, and misery appeared to be compounded. He screamed loudly and threw himself into his mother's arms, sobbing uncontrollably. It was almost impossible to reassure or comfort him. It seemed clear that the father's repeated failure to materialize was leading to severe anxiety with many depressive components. This was epitomized by the untimely intrusion at the crucial evening hour. The child's distress rapidly disappeared after his father returned, and he soon re-established his confident positive relationship.

The second illustration indicates a relatively greater capacity to tolerate separation and possible loss integral to the capacity to tolerate depressive affect. It occurred in almost identical circumstances. This child too showed little overt distress during the day. His sleep, however, had become disturbed and he showed clear indications of distress and anxiety during his wakeful periods. As in the first example, a friend came to pay a visit. As this friend, who resembled the child's father in many ways, entered the room, the child's face lit up in ecstasy. At first glance he had apparently assumed that his father had returned. As the friend approached, he recognized that this was not the case. Severe disappointment and obvious distress showed on his face. He almost burst into tears—his struggle was apparent both to his mother and to the friend. In a few minutes, however, he turned to the friend with an expression of resignation and friendliness, as if to say: 'You aren't the one I want, but I know you. It isn't your fault; you're still a friend, and I'll make the best of an unhappy situation.' This child, although his persistent nocturnal disturbances gave evidence of continued anxious distress, had nevertheless proceeded further towards mastering the limitations of reality than the first little boy, who could only burst into uncontrollable rage and despair when confronted by a parallel situation.

We should note that these two examples, like Freud's (1920), illustrate reactions, in the second year of life, to separation contingent on the previous achievement of individualized personal relationships. Neither of these children was in any way deprived of continued loving care in the absence of the father. Both the anxiety and the sadness depended on an established, essentially positive, specific object relationship. The reaction of the first child, who expressed his distress mainly as explosive rage with acute anxiety, might be described as a time-limited, all-or-nothing response. He perceived the visitor who was not his father as entirely negative and therefore totally rejected him. The second child, in contrast, appears to have made a decisive further step. He was able to make a comparison, to show his disappointment, but nevertheless to turn actively towards the substitute in a friendly, realistic manner. His reaction was not total; he neither relinquished his wish nor denied his longing. He did not reject the substitute, nor did he accept him as a totally adequate replacement.

Both these children, in short, had reached a level of development at which self-object differentiation and a capacity for genuine object relations had been acquired. Both manifested distress in a situation of separation and threatened loss. In both cases the painful affect included components of anxiety and depression. The qualitative difference between the incidents described, however, is fundamental to this discussion. The first little boy showed no observable capacity to contain or to master painful emotions. The second, though he indicated comparable distress in a sleep disturbance, made a recognizable effort in his waking life to accept the painful reality that could not be modified. He had, in addition, initiated the essential developmental step that follows passive acceptance of the inevitable. He made active efforts to relate to a new available object, despite his continued longing for the old.

Neither of these examples is unusual. They are characteristic of the behaviour of pre-oedipal children whose earliest development has been, on the whole, satisfactory. Such children should be differentiated from young babies who have not yet established individualized object relationships. They should also be differentiated from persons of any age whose history and symptomatology suggest sustained inability to recognize and experience genuine unhappiness or depression. Serious psychological disorders of childhood and later life derive from developmental failure which limits the capacity for positive object relations. Furthermore, positive gains in the area of object relations are accompanied by the emergence of sadness and depression in the treatment of severe personality disorders and the psychoses. Pessimism in respect of potential capacities in this area may be a major factor in formulating a poor prognosis for intensive psychotherapy.

The quotation from Chapter 3 referred to problems relevant to the earliest period of ego development. These generally concern factors influencing the capacity to become depressed. They are less directly related to the current discussion than are later factors which affect tolerance and mastery of depression once the capacity to experience painful affect has been achieved. The qualitative difference in the responses of the two little boys illustrates the nature of the developmental step involved. Achievement of the type of response illustrated by the second appears to be essential both for the passive tolerance of inevitable depression and for subsequent optimal active adaptation. Such tolerance has already been compared to Max Schur's concept (1953) of controlled anxiety.

Let us assume for the sake of discussion that the combination of anxiety, rage, and desperation shown by the first little boy represents a response characteristic of an early stage of development. Self-object differentiation, an object relationship and the capacity for early ego identification have been achieved. Neither the sense of personal identity nor the capacity to maintain it has been securely established. Continued absence of an important object, therefore, presents a vital threat to which the child responds with anxiety and rage. Such behaviour, although disturbing, need not lead to disastrous or irreversible consequences. In an adult who has not integrated the capacity to contain depressive affect, the same combination may, however, have very different consequences. In short, persons who have not genuinely achieved the developmental tasks that differentiate my first and second illustrations may demonstrate an intolerance of separation, frustration and depression that may lead to loss of control, impairment of reality testing, psychosis, suicide or murder.

To cite a clinical example: A former patient continued for many years to return for emergency help. Although she had been able to make use of the help of other psychiatrists to a limited degree, she had never accepted separation from me as an established reality. As long as she could re-establish contact, even by telephone, she could reverse repeated episodes of acute depression and anxiety without serious regressive behaviour. This patient, however, moved to a part of the world where personal contact was not directly available. After a short time she became anxious and depressed. She sought psychiatric help with no relief. Her mounting symptoms included a combination of anxiety, rage, impulsive behaviour and depression, which became increasingly intolerable. The regressive course of her illness may be indicated by quotations from her letters:

> I've become exceedingly anxious—I become more and more afraid to reach out and so I withdraw—I'm getting worse. I wake up at 5.30 every morning feeling flooded with panic, shaky, scared and weepy—I do less and less, I withdraw more and more, feel more and more helpless. I'm terribly worried—do you think I should return

to the States and be hospitalized? I'm a drag on everyone around me and most unhappy. . . .

Arrangements had in fact been made for the patient to return when she suddenly changed her mind. The trust, which had been apparent in the first letter, had not been sustained. She developed delusional ideas in which her therapist became a persecutor. Her rage, anxiety and incapacity to tolerate depression led to acute overt psychosis and to hospitalization. In a revealing letter she saw her own downfall: 'My troubles are now my fears and fantasies, but I feel like I'm rushing headlong into making them terrible realities.'

Despite considerable evidence of both early developmental failure and subsequent environmental stress, this patient had made substantial progress over many years. However, her adjustment and adaptation, punctuated as it was by periods of acute panic, remained precarious. These panic states typically reversed readily after brief verbal contact. It was only when direct personal communication became impossible that her failure to contain or tolerate separation and helplessness led to serious ego regression and psychotic behaviour. The responses that then emerged were comparable to the reaction of the first little boy. What was short-lived, reversible and within the normal range of infantile behaviour for the child, however, was long-standing, psychotic, and disastrous for the adult. It represented, in effect, a regression of the ego compounded by early developmental failure specifically related to intolerance of relative helplessness, separation, and acceptance of the limitations of reality. As she regressed further, she was no longer able to recognize the subjective basis of her fears. She then lost the capacity for genuine self-object differentiation and reality testing.

I first saw this patient when she was an impulse-ridden, manipulative late adolescent. Although her life situation was difficult and frustrating, she showed neither depressive affect nor a significant capacity to control anxiety. During the course of treatment her acting out diminished, and she was able to contain anxiety to a degree that enabled her partially to resolve a number of important conflicts. She never, however, completed the developmental tasks which determine the capacity to work through the depressive component, essential to termination of treatment. Underlying resentment, anger and a sense of rage persisted, implicitly if not explicitly. It was this crucial failure that maintained a highly ambivalent transference residuum, usually expressed in the most glowing terms. In times of stress, direct communication enabled her to feel accepted and thus to recover her equilibrium. When this proved impossible, she could not contain the underlying negative feelings.

This case history implies possible parallels between developmental phases and ego regression in adult life. The differences, however, should also be emphasized. While transient acute explosions in young children are to be anticipated in the course of normal development, the regressive emergence of related affect in adult life raises varied and controversial questions. This patient, for example, illustrates more than the role of primitive aggression in both depression and delusion formation; her family background and whole life history make it impossible to exclude genetic, constitutional and biological factors, all of which may have been operative at the time of crucial decompensation.

Clearly, this patient, unlike the second little boy, could not initiate the passive acceptance of the inevitable that must precede the mobilization of active adaptive resources. Her response thus illustrates those manifestations of depression that may be compared to anxiety attributable to relative developmental failure. Both her depression and her subsequent further regression indicate continued failure to accomplish the essential developmental task. The response of the second little boy, in contrast, may be described as an infantile prototype of depression as a potentially adaptive experience. One might suggest that the child's overt struggle illustrates the possible signal function of depression proposed in Bibring's comparison of depression and anxiety. The child's disappointment led neither to inhibition nor to prolonged distress. Rather, it served as a stimulus potentially leading to increased adaptation as a result of his ability to respond positively to available sources of gratification.

That this patient was for many years able to obtain relief and thus to avoid serious regression through brief contact with a trusted therapist is not without theoretical and clinical significance. It is probable that continued availability of the therapist represented an indispensable prerequisite for the maintenance of her more mature ego functions. Though she had reached a capacity for object relations comparable to that of the first little boy, she remained unable to make the vital further step which would have enabled her to tolerate loss and frustration without serious regression. It is likely that many patients whose treatment termination poses insuperable problems fall into a comparable clinical category. Their commitment to the therapist involves a relationship hardly definable as a transference neurosis. The very capacity to utilize therapy depends on achieving a better object relationship than had been possible during the crucial developmental period. A critical question in determining whether or not such patients can complete either analysis or therapy revolves around evaluation of the ability to internalize and identify on the basis of this new relationship. Such an evaluation involves the potential to tolerate not only depressive affect but the regressive forms of anxiety that may emerge in the face of threatened loss. In this context the underlying hostility that determined the patient's delusions points to the close relationship between depression and its tolerance and the mastery of aggression. Individuals who cannot achieve final separation may continue to function effectively on the basis of occasional therapeutic interviews. They seldom abuse the relationship, recognizing the continued importance of the therapist as a real person. One such patient with unusual insight cogently remarked: 'Whenever I begin to feel angry with you, I know that I must make an appointment. Otherwise I'll soon get very depressed.'

This adult patient was able to verbalize a distress similar to that shown by the first little boy. Separation from a vitally important object reinforces aggression on the one hand and impairs positive ego identification on the other. The less secure the integration of the latter, the more will real loss or separation be experienced as rejection. Since, in addition, such lack of security is generally attributable to unresolved ambivalence, ego regression in predisposed individuals will inevitably be associated with increased hostility. Inability to tolerate depression may thus be related to circumstances, whether externally or internally determined, which affect basic attributes of the psychic apparatus. Dynamic and economic factors relate to the maintenance or reinforcement of aggression following frustration, rejection or separation. Structural factors involve a shift from positive ego identification to the more negative identification with the aggressor to the emergence of a harsh, sadistic superego. When significant adverse experiences in early childhood have been aggravated by subsequent separation and loss, the capacity for tolerating depression may be rendered seriously and permanently inadequate. Transference, for such patients, must inevitably remain ambivalent and distrustful for extended periods. Their recognition and acceptance of the passive components of an essentially positive relationship frequently entail a narcissistic injury—the renunciation of the illusions of self-sufficiency.

This symptomatology suggests a close link between Bibring's ego-psychological approach, which emphasized narcissistic injury, and the vulnerability to such injury determined by insecure, ambivalent object relationships. The first little boy's responses suggest that his subjective emotions were highly ambivalent. He did not experience the father's absence exclusively as an object loss. He also experienced it as abandonment or rejection, which threatened a narcissistic injury. In the clinical practice of psychotherapy and psychoanalysis, termination of treatment that has not been achieved on the basis of mutual agreement and mutual respect all too frequently constitutes not only or even mainly object loss, but significant, often serious narcissistic injury. Many patients previously in therapy or analysis who develop depression combined with reappearance of earlier neurotic symptomatology are unable to return to their former therapists. In some cases they feel too ashamed to ask for further help, as they had been apparently cured. In others they explicitly express a sense of rejection in respect of the earlier therapeutic relationship. The therapy indicated for patients of this type involves consolidation and reintegration of the achievements of earlier treatment in the setting of a stable relationship that maintains self-esteem. Certain of these patients, like those described above, appear to be genuinely unable to work through a decisive terminal phase of treatment.

While certain seriously predisposed patients may thus be limited in their potential capacity to achieve mature tolerance of depression, there are many individuals whose gross manifest symptomatology may be deceptive in the reverse direction. Substantial success in respect of the developmental task that differentiates the second little boy from the first may be disguised in adult life by manifest symptomatology primarily attributable to instinctual, rather than ego, regression. Such regression, when it initiates symptom formation of an inhibiting and distressing nature, often leads to manifest guilt, shame and loss of self-esteem. Depression may be noted as a major presenting symptom in the initial evaluation of patients suffering from hysterical and obsessional neuroses who are potentially suitable for psychoanalytic treatment. Such patients frequently require and respond to brief preliminary psychotherapy which re-establishes sufficient self-esteem to facilitate positive therapeutic alliance. Their relative vulnerability to depression, however, must be recognized during the course of treatment, since maintenance of therapeutic alliance is a prerequisite to significant progress.

A brief clinical example will illustrate this last point. A childless married woman of twenty-eight sought consultation with the presenting complaint of depression related to her inability to become pregnant, despite considerable gynaecological investigation and active efforts. There had been recent family pressure on her to consider adopting a baby. At the time of initial evaluation this patient appeared to be quite seriously depressed. She expressed ideas of unworthiness, felt that her apparent sterility exposed her as an unsuccessful woman, acknowledged considerable conflict about her feminine role, and repressed guilt and self-reproach concerning her ambivalence. It became clear that she had been handicapped for many years by severe obsessional symptoms. Unless she could perform perfectly any task she undertook, she felt an utter failure. Whenever she accepted positions involving responsibility, she became so caught up in her perfectionism that she went through alternate waves of over-activity and almost complete paralysis. She had been able to profit somewhat from an earlier period of psychotherapy that had terminated before her marriage. Her failure to produce a family, however, had resulted in considerable decompensation, which in turn led to depression, guilt and self-reproach.

Depressive symptomatology so dominated the clinical picture that the possibility of insight therapy seemed remote. The patient showed a good capacity to form a relationship, however. In addition, by the third interview she showed a capacity for self-scrutiny and a sense of humour that had not been evident at the outset. During a brief period of supportive therapy while she took steps to deal with a physical condition that might have interfered with conception, the patient showed steady improvement. Despite the readiness with which she expressed feelings of inadequacy and self-devaluation, she was also able to recognize the grandiosity of her ego-ideal and to attempt to modify the demands she imposed on herself. Within approximately three months this patient had recovered from a depressive symptomatology that represented decompensation of an obsessional neurosis. She was then referred to a colleague, who subsequently reported satisfactory progress towards a traditional psychoanalysis.

The clinical material so far cited, like that which stimulated 'Anxiety and the Capacity to Bear It' (Chapter 3), derives primarily from observations outside the practice of traditional psychoanalysis. Persons who can tolerate this very demanding therapeutic process belong to a category which represents only a small percentage of depressed patients seeking psychological help. A psychoanalytic understanding of depression, however, must include a wide spectrum of psychiatric illness. Such a goal involves the integration of basic concepts derived from psychoanalytic observations. As David Rapaport (1960) proposed in an illuminating and stimulating discussion of psychoanalytic theory, one should differentiate between that part of specific theory that can be validated only within analytic practice and a more general conceptual framework that should ultimately prove verifiable by experiment.

The discussion up to this point deals with an area of investigation between these two extremes. Observations made by the psychoanalytically sophisticated clinician lend themselves to formulation and theoretical discussion within the framework of psychoanalytic metapsychology. In considering the relevance of basic concepts to the broad field of psychiatry one implies a goal integral to Freud's basic orientation. Such broad-based observations not only invite exploration of basic affects, like anxiety and depression, but also facilitate integration of these concepts with more specific analytic formulations concerning sexual as well as ego development. For example, the developmental failures predisposing soldiers to traumatic neuroses necessarily limited discussion to male patients. A comparable premium on lack of fear and denial of potential helplessness has subsequently been encountered more often in the treatment and psychoanalysis of men than of women. In contrast, developmental failures leading to relative incapacity to tolerate depression and separation anxiety have been met far more frequently in female than in male patients. These women too readily acknowledge their feelings of helplessness and passivity. In consequence they are handicapped in establishing mastery, resolution and optimal adaptation.

A brief review of seventy-two patients (forty-two women and thirty men) followed or treated over three years confirmed a previous impression differentiating the developmental failures leading to areas of vulnerability characteristic of men and of women. Of forty-two women, twenty-three complained of depression as a major presenting symptom. Only six of the thirty men mentioned depression at the time of initial evaluation. All but eight of the women developed and expressed depressive affect and separation anxiety during the course of treatment. Only fourteen men acknowledged either depression or manifest separation anxiety without a long period of preliminary treatment.

Eight of the women and sixteen of the men showed considerable intolerance of both depression and anxiety. Only two of these eight women could be regarded as potentially analysable, both active professional women with marked overt penis envy. The other six were, at best, infantile narcissistic character disorders with minimal capacity to tolerate either anxiety or depression. The others were 'as if' personalities—hypomanic, paranoid or overtly schizophrenic. Of the sixteen men, however, only one half were as disturbed as the women who failed to develop overt painful affect. The others were active, obsessional, often counterphobic characters, who were almost all potentially analysable, since the developmental failure was relative and limited. Indeed the character structure of several was comparable to that of many war neurotics before the traumatic experience. Although potentially vulnerable to trauma or significant narcissistic injury, they were not seriously disturbed or in any sense borderline.

The psychoanalytic significance of these empirical findings is suggestive rather than conclusive. Nevertheless, the fact that only six of these thirty male patients revealed manifest or easily elicited depression is worthy of comment. The relatively high number of individuals seeking therapy or analysis for professional rather than therapeutic goals obviously weights this sample to a significant degree. However, comparison between the professional men and women I have seen or treated still reveals considerable disparity regarding the recognition of subjective depressive affect. This sample, moreover, was drawn from a very general psychiatric practice, including at one extreme the professional group already noted, and at the other, patients sufficiently disturbed to require hospitalization. It may therefore be stated with some certainty that in my own recent clinical experience intolerance of recognized depression is not uncommon in the evaluation and initial treatment of potentially analysable male patients. Depressed men, conversely, have fallen on the whole into a group of more disturbed patients. When analysable, they have been passive, dependent characters with significant problems in the area of masculine identification. When more disturbed, they have typically been seen first in a state of decompensation which bore evidence to serious incapacity to tolerate narcissistic injury.

Retrospectively, as already indicated, the large sample of male traumatic neuroses also revealed a relative incapacity in the same area. Their premorbid history typically elicited unawareness of passivity, depression, anxiety and realistic limitations. In the analysis of well-adapted male patients of comparable character structure this relative failure leads to problems in the analytic situation in achieving the degree of passive dependence indispensable to the analytic process. The development and analysis of the transference neurosis involve mobilization and recognition of some depressive affect. During this process psychoanalysis of such patients has frequently revealed defensive character structure attributable to a neurotic solution of the infantile neurosis. This, in essence, reinforced active achievement to the relative exclusion of the passive components of psychic maturity. The developmental tasks which differentiate the two little boys had been successfully initiated in early childhood. Passive acceptance of reality with its depressive implications had, however, been overshadowed by subsequent investment in the active adaptation so often regarded as synonymous with masculinity. Realistic limitations had thus been underestimated, leaving areas of potential vulnerability to narcissistic injury which re-emerged during analysis of the transference neurosis.

The developmental task relevant to the tolerance and mastery of depression is thus to be regarded as dual. It involves, first, tolerated, passive experience of inability to modify a painful existing reality. Equally important, however, is the subsequent adaptation which involves mobilization of appropriate responses to available areas of gratification and achievement. It has so far been suggested that relative failures in respect of the first may lead to an over-development of the second. Though compatible with long periods of successful adaptation, this type of character development nevertheless retains a crucial Achilles heel.

The premium on activity associated with the masculine ego-ideal reinforces throughout the infantile neurosis the second phase of the developmental task. Accordingly, it is hardly surprising that relative intolerance of passivity and depression may be compatible with an analysable transference neurosis. In women the situation is very different. Passivity rather than activity dominates the image of femininity. Problems, therefore, in initiating or completing the second part of the developmental task may be reinforced during the later stages of the infantile neurosis. This may lead to the exaggerated sense of passivity and helplessness basic to female depressive character structure. Sexualization of the passivity associated with the earliest experience often leads to a combination of this character structure with hysterical symptomatology. Most of the women included in this study could develop and tolerate a considerable degree of depression. Their capacity, however, to mobilize ego-acceptable active resources leading to mastery and growth made them vulnerable to ego regression. This often led to manifest intolerance of depression in response to rejection or significant narcissistic injury.

Over-sexualization of both activity and passivity is relevant to our understanding of castration anxiety in men and of penis envy in women. Significant failure in the earlier developmental task leads in both sexes to an intolerance of depression which precludes successful therapeutic analysis. In men, displaced fantasies of omnipotence may place the premium on continued success which often leads to involutional depression. In women, body-phallus identification and fantasies of a hidden magical penis have related, but more ominous, implications. In milder forms, however, successful initiation of both developmental tasks in the pregenital period may subsequently be disguised by conflicts initiated during the phallic and genital stages of the infantile neurosis. Since this group of patients is potentially suitable for therapeutic analysis, its differentiation from the more disturbed group must be regarded as extremely important.

It is implicit in my thesis that the dichotomy passivity–femininity versus activity–masculinity may be highly deceptive. Positive identification with the mother during the pregenital period acts as a stimulus towards independence and autonomy in healthy little girls. It is a common observation that little boys, whose object investment may be greater, are often content to be served by their mothers for a significantly longer period. In little girls, identification with the mother should help rather than hinder the emergence, development and renunciation of passive genital wishes towards the father. When for whatever reason, however, a premium has been placed on active achievement as a means of gaining approval, an underlying, continued passive goal remains. Such a combination may seriously interfere with the development and resolution of the oedipal situation. It may, for example, lead to a defensive reinforcement of penis envy which hides from the outside world an underlying depressive character structure and continued passive needs. Many patients who develop difficult, demanding transference neuroses belong to this group.

The evaluation of penis envy and phallic behaviour presents many complex problems relevant to my subject. In 'Analysis Terminable and Interminable' Freud said:

> At no other point in one's analytic work does one suffer more from an oppressive feeling that all one's repeated efforts have been in vain, and from a suspicion that one has been 'preaching to the winds', than when one is trying to persuade a woman to abandon her wish for a penis on the ground of its being unrealizable. . . . We often have the impression that with the wish for a penis . . . we have . . . reached bedrock, and that thus our activities are at an end. This is probably true, since, for the psychical field, the biological field does in fact play the part of the underlying bedrock (1937, p. 252).

Biological factors, though they represent bedrock in the sense that they are unalterable, do not represent unalterable features of psychic life. Rather, intense penis envy at a phallic level may well be determined by a relative failure to achieve acceptance of reality and genuine object relations during pregenital development. An active, essentially phallic orientation characterizes the pre-oedipal period of genital activity. In both sexes, earlier developmental deficits affecting the acceptance of reality may lead to intensification of this later active level. In girls, intense penis envy during this period may be associated with persistent fantasies of a magical hidden phallus. This may derive from continued failure to perceive, let alone accept, the limitations of reality. Women whose early failure has led to this pathological character formation may never come to the attention of the psychiatrist. They may, in some cases, first be seen when psychosis has become manifest. They may commit suicide. Some of them, though partially analysable, cannot work through a successful terminal process. Where penis envy and a phallic orientation are essentially defensive and motivated by underlying passive wishes for approval, however, the incapacity to tolerate depression derives from a regressive solution of the oedipal situation, which falls within the category of analysable character neuroses. Early developmental failure that results in a relatively unalterable limitation must thus be differentiated from symptomatology and character defences attributable to a regressive solution of the infantile neurosis. This differentiation is equally vital to the understanding of men and women, for it represents a critical factor in determining the potential capacity to work through the terminal stages of psychoanalysis.

Although I have so far illustrated my main points by brief, non-analytic clinical examples, I should now like to illustrate the progressive and adaptive value of depression by material derived from the terminal phases of a successful therapeutic analysis. The patient was a highly intelligent married woman, who had entered analysis with presenting symptoms of a predominantly phobic and hysterical nature. In addition to her symptoms, however, her character structure included defences attributable to intense penis envy and a phallic orientation. On the one hand, there was evidence of an entrenched body-phallus fantasy; on the other, she manifested an unconscious conviction that she possessed a hidden, magical penis that in certain circumstances she could give to an otherwise devalued man, thus endowing him with genital potency. This fantasy was displaced upward and acted out in a number of rather intense intellectual relationships. Early in the analysis she saw the analyst, a woman, predominantly as a prohibiting, threatening mother. Although the patient expressed considerable hostility, she was able to maintain sufficient therapeutic alliance to recognize the pathology of her fantasies and to accept the analyst's essential neutrality with regard to her real life situation.

In addition to her role as mother-surrogate, the analyst, who was married, appeared from an early stage of the analysis as an omnipotent phallic woman, with whom the patient sought to identify at a very primitive level. The patient could accept neither the analyst's real behaviour nor occasional outside information indicating certain areas in which the analyst might be open to criticism or devaluation. Instead, she distorted and denied both her own perceptions and her outside information in order to maintain her fantasy of the analyst's perfection and omnipotence. Finally, in contrast to these two aspects of the transference neurosis, a third gradually emerged. This aspect was for a long time limited to occasional transference dreams, in which the analyst appeared as a tender, maternal figure. For a long time the patient minimized and devalued these feelings. She did not wish to see her analyst either as a woman or as a mother. This seriously threatened her intense devaluation of femininity and motherhood. It also disclosed her deep fear of an overprotective, dominating mother, from whom she would not be able to separate. Changes in this respect first appeared in relation to her own children. For the first time she experienced positive maternal feelings and recognized less need to dominate and control, and displayed a greater capacity to encourage her children's independent development. Meanwhile, her relationship with her husband improved, mainly in the total family situation.

She had, however, given up neither her penis envy nor her underlying fantasy that she had a penis. Her acting out had diminished, mainly as a means of pleasing and conciliating her analyst. In spite of growing recognition that the analyst was not really an omnipotent phallic figure, the patient continued in the transference neurosis to regard her predominantly in this role. She responded to interpretations indicating that she had never, in fact, possessed a hidden penis by projecting omnipotence on to the analyst, whom she regarded for a time as the primary castrator. This aspect of the transference neurosis corresponded closely to her childhood situation. Her mother had in fact been a powerful castrating figure; her father, a dependent, passive, physically incapacitated man.

A sequence of events that occurred at this juncture marked a milestone in her analysis. She had been helping her daughter with her homework and had struggled against her inclination either to demand too much or to do the child's work for her. She had succeeded in showing the little girl certain principles and then had left her to do the work. She felt, however, that she had been rather strict and impatient in the process. Later in the evening she watched two television programmes with her daughter. The first was a dramatization of the life of Helen Keller which has since become well known as the play *The Miracle Worker*. During this programme the mother had been struck by Miss Sullivan's approach to her charge. Helen Keller's concerned and over-protective parents had indulged her and allowed her unlimited gratification. Miss Sullivan introduced discipline and limitations from the outset. At the same time she tried to communicate with the child by means of the manual alphabet. At first the patient identified with Helen Keller, resenting the imposed limitations and demands. Then came the scene in which Helen Keller first understood the meaning of the word 'water'—responding not only with excitement and eagerness to learn more, but also showing for the first time spontaneous affection for her teacher. To the patient there was an intimate connection between the imposition of limitations on the one hand, and the acquisition of skill, understanding and the capacity for object relations on the other. Tears came into her eyes, and she said to herself: 'This is what the analyst means. In order to grow up, I have to accept certain negatives as part of reality.' This insight was reinforced by the second programme, during which her daughter, towards whom she felt she had been somewhat harsh and demanding, came and sat on her lap, showing an affection and gratitude that reminded her of Helen Keller's response to Annie Sullivan.

The second programme, based on Oscar Wilde's fairy tale *The Happy Prince*, concerned a prince, who throughout his life had been protected from all contact with any experience of evil and suffering. After his death he was turned into a statue that stood on a pedestal high enough to give a view over the walls of the palace to the suffering world outside. The statue's eyes overflowed with tears, and it requested a bird to give to the needy the prince's clothes, jewels, eyes and, finally, his heart. In the end the statue was denuded, and the bird dead. Again the patient was moved to tears, seeing clearly, as she reported next day, that reality is not all one way or the other. Negatives should be accepted, and one should not be dominated by fantasy. The prince, who knew only gratification, had to destroy himself when he met evil. She, too, had seen negatives as too overwhelming to surmount. In the past she had avoided and repressed certain wishes that would have confronted her with her own limitations, in particular the lack of a real penis. Acceptance of reality meant a positive acknowledgement of the differences between men and women. True, she had no penis. She had, however, real children and a real husband. Although they imposed certain limitations and unpleasant duties, they also gave real gratifications. She then associated to a recent incident in respect of a political organization of a type that would previously have aroused her rivalry with men. She had not felt competitive, but instead had been aware of the value of certain qualifications she had as a woman and a mother.

Although she expressed this material mainly in terms of a general attitude towards reality, there was in the weeks that followed considerable evidence of a qualitative change in the therapeutic alliance. Associations to a dream, for example, showed that she was now able to face the possibility that she might disagree with or criticize the analyst without undue anxiety. For the first time she was able to feel that the analyst might not be perfect, might have problems and limitations of her own, but at the same time might avoid letting these problems interfere with the analytic situation or her relationship with the patient. She no longer denied or distorted her information, nor did she feel unduly distressed at reporting it in analysis. The qualitative change was further confirmed following an occasion on which the patient heard the analyst speak in public. She was able for the first time to see the analyst as a real person who did not, as a matter of fact, very closely resemble her previously fantasied transference picture. While she identified with certain of the analyst's interests and ideas, she was still aware of important individual differences and was therefore able to maintain a sense of her own separate identity. Her attitude in this terminal stage of analysis illustrated certain aspects of therapeutic alliance. She could now identify at a mature level with the analyst's approach to the analytic task. Yet it was abundantly clear that this capacity depended at its deepest levels on an object relationship that recognized delineation of ego boundaries.

As her analysis proceeded towards definite termination the patient experienced increased conflict between pleasure over her increased autonomy and anxiety concerning revived dependent wishes. This depressive anxiety was closely linked to some realistic concern about her physical health. She recognized that severe illness in the past had frequently led to regression to earlier ambivalent patterns in which omnipotent fantasies alternated with angry, helpless dependence. She recalled her helpless anxiety and rage when, after the birth of her first child, her mother had departed to care for one of her sisters. That she was nearing termination had become clear when she had almost forgotten a regular analytic hour because of a pleasant invitation. This had made her aware of an increasing wish for greater freedom, which at first she viewed with considerable pleasure. The next day, however, she reported two nightmares so severe that she had called out in her sleep. The two dreams were very similar. In the first, one of her children was going blind. She felt anxious and frustrated, mainly concerned with her dread of responsibility for a helpless burden. In the second, her dog had sustained injuries not severe enough to kill him but so incapacitating that, like the child, he would become completely dependent on her. In her associations she described some anger at the child's stubborn, infantile behaviour the night before. She had felt angry that her daughter was not so independent as she herself had been in early childhood. She recalled an incident when she had stayed out for dinner without telling her parents and had been surprised at their anger. Now suddenly she realized that she had stayed away in order to get attention, even if negative. Although superficially independent, she had been accident-prone and had had many serious illnesses; her mother had been attentive only when she was sick. She had had many suitors, but she had married the only one who would take her a long way from home. She resented her sister's continued dependence on the mother. As she went on talking she became more and more aware of her own ambivalence towards the growing independence of her children. She was afraid that she might damage them by being either rejecting or over-protective. But she recognized that her current feelings towards them really derived from the transference situation and the ambivalence of her own increasing wish for autonomy and independence.

The material so far reported indicates the conflict characteristic of the type of anxiety I have described as depressive. As the patient increasingly mastered this anxiety, she began to experience a more contained type of depressive affect. In this phase she reported another dream. She dreamed that she had undergone an operation—it didn't hurt—and something had been removed. It seemed to have a cylindrical shape. The startling thing was that she did not feel as if anything had changed or been taken out. Her associations led to a close friend who, despite crippling illness, had remained essentially the same person. She no longer felt terrified at the thought of illness or operation, having recognized that she could remain the same person even if something were taken away. She then said, with a start of recognition, that even if she realized that something had never been there, she could still be a whole person. She thus no longer felt so threatened by many of the things that had previously worried her so much. She particularly emphasized attitudes towards illness, damage and, finally, separation

This dream and her associations indicate an acceptance of reality in respect of penis envy which touches on Freud's remarks (1937). We should also note, however, that acceptance of realistic limitations was intimately related to the emergence of contained depressive affect concerned with imminent separation and object loss. In my experience I have regarded no analysis as successfully terminated in which comparable depressive emotions have not been experienced and mastered. Termination of analysis may thus be compared with the type of response shown by the second little boy. It includes some measure of sorrow and renunciation. It also includes acceptance of the inevitable.

Finally, it is an essential prerequisite to the active adaptive capacity to utilize available resources essential for the future mastery of inevitable frustration and loss.

The considerations raised in this chapter are entirely compatible with the brilliant blueprints made half a century ago by Freud (1917), Abraham (1924) and others. The capacity to become depressed is initiated during the oral phase of development. Experiences relevant to the emergence of subjective depression, related anxiety and early attempts at mastery occur before the onset of the genital oedipal situation. Of the matter of instinctual points of fixation and the content of unconscious fantasy, little has been said in this chapter. Depression, however, has been defined as a basic ego state. One major ego function concerns recognition and acceptance of reality. This ego function was described by Freud long before the structural hypothesis was explicitly formulated. He said:

> While the ego goes through its transformation from a *pleasure-ego* into a *reality-ego*, the sexual instincts undergo the changes that lead them from their original auto-erotism through various intermediate phases to object-love in the service of procreation. If we are right in thinking that each step in these two courses of development may become the site of a disposition to later neurotic illness, it is plausible to suppose that the form taken by the subsequent illness . . . will depend on the particular phase of the development of the ego and of the libido in which the dispositional inhibition of development has occurred. Thus unexpected significance attaches to the chronological features of the two developments (which have not yet been studied), and to possible variations in their synchronization (1911, p. 224 f.).

Structural and dynamic attributes of the psychic apparatus need not, as Freud hinted, necessarily develop concurrently or harmoniously. For example, it was the younger of the two little boys who showed the more mature ego capacity to accept reality. This child's earlier development and subsequent history suggest economic differences in respect of primitive aggressive instinctual energy and earlier onset of a capacity to tolerate delay and frustration. It may be suggested, therefore, that we should differentiate between instinctual fixation that may determine the content of adult symptomatology and partial or significant failure in the initiation and integration of basic ego functions. Such failures may determine vulnerability to ego regression in response to depression and the related primitive anxiety that cannot be tolerated or contained.

Acute separation anxiety and explosive rage often precede the emergence of genuine sadness or depression. This affect marks the first decisive step towards achieving the passive component of psychic maturity. Partial failure in this area may subsequently be overshadowed by activity and external adaptation. Substantial success leads to the capacity to contain or tolerate depression without serious ego regression. The capacity to regress in the service of the ego is also contingent on the completion of the developmental task. Once achieved, however, passive acceptance must be followed by the active mastery which facilitates the development of object relations, learning and ultimately the capacity for happiness.

No matter how great the opportunities for passive gratification and active achievement, renunciation and loss are essential to human experience. Mature, passive acceptance of the inevitable thus remains a sustained prerequisite to the remobilization of available adaptive resources at all times. While failure in this vital area may be consistent with long periods of successful adaptation, it represents a serious potential vulnerability that becomes increasingly relevant in the later years of life, when experiences of loss, grief and frustration are not to be avoided. In his conclusion to *Childhood and Society* (1950) Erik Erikson said: 'Healthy children will not fear life if their parents have integrity enough not to fear death.' I submit that healthy children who do not fear life—in spite of subjective awareness of its limitations—will become adults with integrity enough not to fear death.

7

CONCEPT AND CONTENT IN PSYCHOANALYTIC THEORY[1]

(1956)

The relation between theory and practice is a central problem in the development of every branch of science. In the physical sciences, it is relatively easy to make a clear distinction between the objective data which lead to theoretical hypotheses and the objective experiments which confirm those hypotheses. With the growth of psychoanalytic thought and its expansion not only to the problems of clinical psychiatry, but to the related fields of anthropology, social relations and general psychology, there is inevitably increasing interest in similar methods of validation. In psychoanalysis, however, even more than in the other social sciences, both the lack of concrete objective data and the relative difficulty of repeating observational situations lead to special problems in objective validation. In addition, however, to this problem, which is well recognized in all social sciences, the development of psychoanalysis is a special case in that it presents inherent difficulties in making a clear distinction not only between theory and practice, but also between theoretical hypotheses based on the interpretation of specific content, and theoretical hypotheses of a more general abstract nature concerning the structure and function of the mental apparatus itself. The development and validation of our science, in short, would appear to involve at least a threefold task; namely, first, the collection of clinical data; second, evaluation of such clinical data, leading to theories based on the content or meaning of the data; and third, general concepts of an abstract nature deduced from these formulations.

The development of psychoanalytic knowledge has from the

[1] First published, under the title 'An Approach to the Relation between Concept and Content in Psychoanalytic Theory', in *Psychoanal. Study Child* (1956), 11.

outset been concerned with ever deeper and more penetrating investigation into the specific content of the unconscious mind, into the nature of unconscious fantasies, into the various mechanisms by means of which unconscious impulses are modified and controlled, and into the specific situations, both external and internal, which can be related to the development of the ego and the sense of reality. The correlation of the findings of different workers in respect of these problems has been a main preoccupation of psychoanalytic research. It would probably be correct to say that the general body of knowledge derived from these investigations into the content of the unconscious mind has in a number of respects reached a stage where formulations of a general nature have been incorporated into our theoretical framework. The different stages of libidinal development, the specific content of oedipal fantasies, and the essential nature of the definitive superego, for example, have been formulated in theoretical terms based largely on interpretation of content. In addition to this type of theoretical formulation one must also consider another set of deductions which have been proposed as the basis for a general theoretical framework. This aspect of theory is not concerned primarily with the specific content of the unconscious mind, but rather with abstract conceptual formulations which are capable of subsuming the infinite complexities of other findings of a more specific meaningful nature.

The problem with which this chapter is concerned, it will be seen, is the general problem of validation as it relates to the correlation of observed clinical facts with theoretical postulates. Some qualifications must, however, be made. In the first place, the question of objective validation *per se* is not under consideration. In the second place, this chapter will attempt to concentrate mainly on the relation, within the theoretical framework, between formulations concerned with interpretation of content and abstract deductions of a general nature. Certain generally accepted analytic hypotheses, mainly concerned with discovering of content or meaning, form an integral part of psychoanalytic theory. Other basic premises, in contrast, refer to more general abstract concepts concerning, for example, the structure and function of the psychic apparatus, general instinct theory, and fundamental views regarding the nature of anxiety.

Freud's 'Interpretation of Dreams' (1900) might be regarded

as the model for the differentiation of these two aspects of psychoanalytic theory. The first six chapters of that book come mainly under the heading of content; the seventh chapter is concerned with concept. It would be fair to say that, in the earlier chapters, Freud is primarily concerned with a clinical approach to dream material. From associations and the resistances thereto, he elucidates not only the latent meaning, or content, of the dream, but the various specific mechanisms by means of which the latent content is disguised and distorted in the manifest dream structure. He is able, by means of specific meaningful illustrations, to demonstrate the underlying meaning of the dream and is also able to relate the dream work to the nature and to the content of the unconscious mind. In the seventh chapter, in contrast, he attempts to draw from this essentially concrete material general deductions as to the nature of the psychic apparatus which could account for his specific meaningful findings. Here, his approach is conceptual and abstract rather than meaningful in terms of the specific content of unconscious wishes or conflicts. In the earlier parts of the book, for example, he refers to the specific sexual nature of repressed material and illustrates in a number of cases the underlying oedipal conflict. The final chapter of the book, on the other hand, is not concerned primarily with the meaning of the psychic or instinctual energy concerned, but formulates a hypothesis of the *structure* of psychic apparatus which modifies and controls instinctual energy, whatever its source.

These brief remarks should indicate both the nature of contrast under consideration, and the difficulty in drawing rigid lines of demarcation. For example, from clinical observations of resistance and from his elucidation of its cause, Freud deduced the existence of the mechanism of repression. This was a theoretical concept with manifold implications familiar to all of us. At the same time, Freud also gave definite indications as to the nature of the repressed, which he at the time mainly limited to repressed sexual wishes at a genital level. The concept of repression is a general concept which has altered very little in its fundamental meaning since Freud first defined it, and it remains a concept basic to current psychoanalytic theory. With regard to content, we can also still agree as to Freud's correct elucidation of the importance of the oedipal conflict as an essential feature of the content of the repressed. Further work and deeper investigation have shown that this early formulation, although correct, was by no means exhaustive so that we would now regard pregenital conflicts antedating the genital oedipal situation as being potentially susceptible to repression. This expansion of content, however, in no way affects the validity of the original concept and only indicates, to my mind, the importance of distinguishing between these two approaches.

With regard to repression, alteration and expansion of our knowledge have not made necessary any radical alteration of basic concepts, for increased knowledge of the content of the repressed has not invalidated the concept of repression; our expanded knowledge of the other mechanisms of defence, as Anna Freud (1936) has shown so clearly, although it has enriched has not invalidated the concept of repression. In his earliest formulations, however, Freud made other tentative suggestions of a conceptual nature which have been vitally affected by later findings regarding content.

To give an example from Freud's own work: in his early formulations of instinct theory, he suggested a dichotomy between the sexual and the ego instincts. This dichotomy was originally based on the hypothesis that repression and the related defence mechanisms were set up by the ego or self-preservative instincts in opposition to dangers threatened by the sexual instincts. According to this formulation, mental conflict was ascribed to opposition between these two drives. Anxiety appeared as a result of the repression enforced by the ego instincts. Later, however, his investigation of the content of the fantasies and delusions of psychotic patients, combined with a number of observations of the traumatic war neuroses, indicated that the original dichotomy he had postulated between libido and the ego instincts could not account for the investment of the ego itself with libido, so clearly revealed in these and allied conditions. As a result of these observations, he recognized that it was necessary to alter his conception of the nature of the instincts. Further investigation as to the nature of anxiety, moreover, revealed that anxiety could function as a cause of repression or motive for defence, a development which complicated his earlier concept of anxiety as the product of instinctual tension and frustration. The subsequent modification of his earlier conceptual framework, both with regard to the nature of the basic instincts and with regard to anxiety as a motive for defence, initiated the development of a structural approach with its manifold implications for modern ego psychology.

It is clear, in following the development of Freud's theoretical work and correlating it with contemporary clinical findings of other pioneers in our field, that modifications of basic concepts have been, with one or two exceptions, closely related to the expansion of analytic knowledge regarding content. It was one of the special qualities of Freud's genius to combine in a unique manner intuitive understanding of the meaning of unconscious content with a capacity for conceptual deduction of a general abstract nature. He was able to recognize spontaneously the meaning of symbols, the manifold and startling manifestations of unconscious mental life and to interpret specific conflicts arising in the analytic situation. On the other hand, he never lost sight of the general, abstract or conceptual implications of his findings. It is desirable that every theoretical contribution to psychoanalytic thought should be oriented both to its implications with regard to content, and also to its conceptual significance. This type of correlation is, however, probably one of the most difficult tasks, not only in psychoanalysis but in psychological thought as a whole. As Marjorie Brierley states in this connection:

> There may be only one event, the psychological event, but there are very definitely two different methods of . . . approaching it. As T. H. Pear (1948) says, 'Psychologists . . . are often distinguished by the emphasis, theoretical and practical, which they place on one of two aims: the discovery of general laws of mind, or the description and understanding of the unique and undivided personality.' The results of both approaches have to be correlated, and can be used to correct each other. At the present stage of thinking development, the distinction between them is readily lost and we should gain by choosing words which help to keep the difference clear (1951, p. 94).

The ability to maintain this distinction depends on a capacity to separate the concrete from the abstract, which is extremely difficult in a science, the nature of which is essentially so subjective. Even Freud occasionally fell into the error of couching his theoretical propositions in too concrete terms. The first difficulty, therefore, in maintaining a clear distinction between concept and content can be attributed to the nature of the material with which we are dealing. As Hartmann, Kris and Loewenstein (1946) have said, 'Our reformulation shows that not the concepts which Freud introduces are anthropomorphic, but that the clinical facts he studied and described lead us to understand what part anthropomorphism plays in introspective thinking.' In spite of this difficulty, which is inherent in our material, it can probably be agreed that during the early stages of development of psychoanalytic knowledge and theory the practice and the science of psychoanalysis were inevitably so closely interwoven that almost without exception every new clinical discovery could be readily considered in terms of its theoretical implications. With the vast expansion of knowledge, clinical experience and literature, however, there has tended to be an increasing separation between those who are primarily interested in utilizing clinical material to enrich our understanding of the content of the unconscious, and those who are predominantly concerned with the clarification of psychoanalytic theory. Of recent years, there have been other analytic thinkers with at least Freud's capacity for abstract conceptual thinking, leading to valuable contributions, reformulating certain basic concepts, using the model set up by Freud (1900) in 'The Interpretation of Dreams' and modifying it in the light of a more structural approach. Many of these papers have, however, been of an extremely abstract nature, leaving to the reader the burden of interpolating the significance of general hypotheses in terms of specific content. In spite of the very great value of such formulations couched in general abstract terms, there is, here, a potential danger that these formulations might be compatible with divergent interpretations of clinical material. This will be considered below in relation to Melanie Klein's work.

On the one hand then, there have been recent valuable contributions to our conceptual thinking which have been more or less divorced from specific content. On the other hand, there have been many gifted analysts with a deep understanding of the unconscious mental life of their patients, who have presented findings which to a greater or lesser extent have been correlated with the general body of psychoanalytic knowledge. In particular, there have been many valuable contributions proposing modifications and reformulations of our present views concerning the nature and meaning of conflict situations in the early months of life. Among these contributions, for example, one must include the work of René Spitz (1946), Edith Jacobson (1946), Margaret Mahler (1952), Bertram Lewin (1950), Beata Rank (1949), Phyllis Greenacre (1952) and Melanie Klein (1935, 1948). The formulations some of these writers have put forward are couched in general terms, but nevertheless should be regarded on the whole as interpretation of content rather than conceptual propositions. Edith Jacobson (1953), for example, in her important investigation of the metapsychology of depression and schizophrenia, has made suggestions regarding self-representation and object-representation and the regressive reanimation of parental images in pathological situations. Greenacre (1952) has correlated her analytic reconstructions with certain objective observations and investigations of infantile behaviour. She clearly indicates the possible pathological implications of excessive stimulation and severe frustration for future development of the ego and of the capacity to deal with anxiety. Spitz (1945, 1946) has made detailed observations of infants under institutional conditions and has drawn some general deductions as to the importance of the object relations in early infancy. Beata Rank (1949), from detailed analytic investigation of certain groups of abnormal children, has also drawn general deductions regarding the role of aggression and the fateful result of maternal deprivation. To discuss the conceptual implications of all of this valuable work would take us far afield. At this point it may be well to consider the contributions of the most controversial of these writers, Melanie Klein, in order to indicate in some detail the relation of concept to content in her work, and to correlate in certain respects some of her views with more recent reformulations of basic concepts. The aim here is not to give an exhaustive discussion of all of Melanie Klein's work (which has been ably criticized by Robert Waelder (1937), Edward Bibring (1947), Edward Glover (1945) and Marjorie Brierley (1951)) but to select certain aspects particularly related to the topic under discussion.

In many ways, Melanie Klein's work is eminently suitable for this purpose. In the first place, many of the difficulties and problems raised by her theoretical formulations may be at least partially attributed to an inadequate distinction between observations enriching our knowledge of content and conceptual deductions as to the theoretical implications of these findings. Her work thus illustrates the vital importance of maintaining this differentiation in the development of psychoanalytic theory. In the second place, the overwhelming emphasis in Melanie Klein's work on unconscious fantasy as the mental expression of instinct; on concrete and specific fantasies as active from the dawn of life; on the ego as entirely derived from the id, marks an extreme contrast to the abstract conceptual approach exemplified by Heinz Hartmann (1950) and David Rapaport (1967) who, following on the whole Freud's approach in the last chapter of 'The Interpretation of Dreams' (1900), attempt to make general formulations relatively divorced from meaningful content. It should be possible, by discussing and comparing both the value and the possible disadvantages of these two extremes, to indicate general problems which not only concern these specific contributors but also illustrate the relationship here postulated between concept and content in the development of psychoanalytic theory.

From clinical observations derived from analyses of young children and later from analyses of borderline patients and psychotics, Melanie Klein (1932) became aware earlier than most analysts of the importance of aggression in early mental development. Moreover, from the same sources, she also recognized that depressive tendencies were far more important in the early stages of development than had previously been suspected. It would seem probable that the fact that Melanie Klein was a pupil of Abraham played some role in her search for and discovery of the importance of introjective mechanisms in these depressive aspects of early life. The close relationship between introjection and projection has long been recognized. In his discussion, moreover, of the metapsychology of psychotic depression, Abraham (1924) had clearly indicated the important role in the genesis of depressive states of objects introjected in an ambivalent or hostile manner. Melanie Klein (1932), applying these concepts to her analysis of young children, brought together her clinical observation of animistic fantasies of both a projective and introjective nature, and her increasing conviction of the important role of aggression in the development of anxiety. She reached the conclusion that the infant's life is dominated by alternating processes of introjection and projection, caused by the infant's need to overcome anxiety involving his aggressive fantasies, chiefly through the development of libido and its fusion with aggression. At the same time, however, this general proposition was amplified by increasing material regarding the specific nature of the fantasies by means of which these processes were expressed. She became increasingly convinced, from her clinical observations of young children, that there was strong evidence suggesting that these primitive fantasies contained elements of an oedipal conflict at a period far antedating the classical oedipal situation. This, she felt, suggested that the type of depression which she attributed to the early months of life could be compared in all essential respects with the structure of depression in the post-oedipal period as described by Abraham (1924).

In other words, she did not feel that her findings necessitated any alteration of the analytic hypothesis that depression was related to a pathological relationship between superego and ego, even though the depression antedated the time usually ascribed to superego development. Pushing her investigations to an ever earlier period, she concluded that the depressive position of infancy represented a relatively advanced stage of development related to the acquisition of true or whole object relationship. Antedating this period, she suggested the infant's mental life was dominated by his anxiety with regard to his own aggressive impulses, proposing that his projection of these impulses on to the outside world could be described as essentially paranoid. During this early period, moreover, she postulated the existence of oedipal fantasies including genital impulses which she considered to be present from a very early period of life. Her assumption in this connection appeared to imply the existence of inborn, innate fantasies of an oedipal nature with some knowledge from the earliest days of life of the difference between the sexes, the relationship between the parents and the way in which babies are born.

To consider, briefly, in a preliminary fashion some of the controversial aspects of her point of view, without at present taking up in detail their full significance, her assumption that anxiety is ultimately attributable to the aggressive impulse is open to question on clinical grounds alone. Secondly, it is difficult to elucidate the evidence on which Melanie Klein (1932, 1948) bases her conviction that oedipal conflicts arise so early in life. As Marjorie Brierley has noted:

> . . . the ages given for the actual beginning of treatment [over two years of age in every case] appear to justify the view that the 'clinical evidence' for Melanie Klein's reconstruction of the first year is mainly inference from conditions observed at later ages . . . [and is] the basis of numerous contentions that Melanie Klein reads back into early development conditions that obtain only in later stages (1951, p. 59).

The problem in this respect is a complex one. On the one hand, there is increasing evidence, as indicated, for example, by Phyllis Greenacre's work (1952), as to the frequent occurrence of genital activity in the early months of life, particularly under conditions of overstimulation or frustration. That such activity should be related to the development of the oedipal conflict is undoubted. Most analysts, however, feel that such premature genital activity leads to distortion, both in the development of early object relationships and to pathological variations of the later true oedipal conflict. It is, in general, considered unlikely that oedipal fantasies of the type postulated by Melanie Klein are compatible with the general level of maturation at the period to which she ascribes them. The fantasies themselves, however, described by Melanie Klein (1932) have been confirmed by Edith Jacobson (1946), Beata Rank (1949) and others, but ascribed to regressive reanimation of earlier less specific fantasies rather than interpreted as evidence of the occurrence of such fantasies at the earlier period itself.

It may be helpful at this point to indicate the very real importance of certain of Melanie Klein's observations.

(1) Her recognition of the important role of aggression in early mental life has been confirmed by many other analytic observers.

(2) Her recognition of the importance of object relations, in particular, the importance of the early mother–child relationship in helping the child to master its aggressive anxieties and fantasies, has also been widely confirmed by a number of child analysts.

(3) The relationship of difficulties in connection with the

mother to early depressive tendencies has also been indicated by other workers. Here one might mention specifically the work of René Spitz (1946) in New York and of Beata Rank and her co-workers in Boston (Rank, 1949; Rank and MacNaughton, 1950).

(4) Melanie Klein's early recognition of the role of anxiety as a spur to development and of the part played by symbol formation in early play, in early fantasy and the development of sublimation is of the utmost importance.

From the point of view, therefore, of depth of clinical observations, there is no doubt that Melanie Klein has made very valuable contributions to our knowledge. It is noteworthy, however, that the contributions which appear to be most acceptable and which could be most easily integrated into the general conceptual framework of analytic theory come under the heading of content rather than concept. Through her recognition of the role of aggression and of introjective and projective mechanisms, Melanie Klein has enriched our knowledge of early fantasy life and has shown the derivation, from an early period of life, though possibly not as early as she suggests, of many of the animistic anxiety-provoking fantasies and delusions so familiar to us in the mental status of psychotic patients.

These remarks may now be amplified by more detailed consideration of the relation between Melanie Klein's (1948) views on aggression, first to the recent papers of Hartmann, Kris and Loewenstein (1949) and Anna Freud (1949), and second, to Freud's theory of the death instinct (1920). It may thus be possible to illustrate the need to distinguish between propositions regarding content and those regarding fundamental conceptual orientation, and also to indicate the degree to which abstract formulations of fundamental concept may be compatible with essentially divergent interpretations of content. This point may first be illustrated by specific reference to the paper by Hartmann, Kris and Loewenstein (1949), 'Notes on the Theory of Aggression', to show how closely the abstract concepts put forward in this paper may be correlated with many of Melanie Klein's propositions.

As already indicated, Melanie Klein, in her analyses of disturbed children and psychotics, became increasingly aware of the importance of aggressive fantasies and the profound anxieties to which they gave rise. She recognized how the conflict between love and hate, and resultant difficulties in achieving a good object relationship, played a crucial role in early development. These points have been discussed earlier in Chapter 5. At this point, the questions previously discussed as to her timing of these conflicts will not be treated, nor at this juncture is it to the point to give detailed discussion as to whether the aggressive instincts are, in the first instance, directed towards the self or the outside world. In this connection, it is noted that Hartmann, Kris and Loewenstein (1949), like Anna Freud (1949) in her paper on this subject, also avoid discussion of this aspect and consider the types of conflict aroused by aggression and the various means by which the aims of aggression are modified. Here, they suggest four main types of conflict: (1) Aggression and libido may be involved in conflict when the cathexis of both drives is vested in the same object (instinctual conflict). (2) The reaction of the object to attempts at completion of aggressive acts may endanger the individual (conflict with reality). (3) This danger may be anticipated by the ego which is in part already identified with the object, and the ego may be opposed to the completion of aggressive acts (structural conflict involving the ego). (4) The conflict may involve moral values (structural conflict involving the superego).

I should like to take up these general conceptual statements in relation to Melanie Klein's formulations.

(1) Hartmann, Kris and Loewenstein (1949) referred to instinctual conflict when aggression and libido are directed towards the same object. They ascribe the relation of object development to fusion of aggression and libido and note the importance of libido development for the creation of good object relations. Melanie Klein makes many statements which are theoretically compatible with this formulation. Ignoring for the moment the degree to which she attributes early anxiety to the death instinct, she also notes the relation of ambivalence to instinctual conflict, and her concept of the depressive position and its mastery makes explicit reference to a development of libido, which in satisfactory development should lead to a creation of good object relations, threatened though they may be by the continued activity of aggression and its concomitant anxiety.

(2) Hartmann, Kris and Loewenstein (1949) consider, under

the heading conflict with reality, dangers which may arise as a result of aggressive acts, which precipitate retaliation on the part of the object. They do not clearly state how far this conflict with reality should be regarded as a real danger and how far the fears of retaliation may be limited to the realm of fantasy. They take into account, however, the possibility that the infant may respond to retaliatory or hostile impulses of which the object may be unconscious, so that their work here may be correlated not only with the work of Melanie Klein, but with Beata Rank's proposals regarding the source of many early traumatic situations. While, therefore, Melanie Klein's greater preoccupation with the role of instinctual conflict and of internal objects colours her presentation of early anxiety situation in relation to their internal sources, there does not appear to be any serious conceptual conflict between her views and those of Hartmann, Kris and Loewenstein. Both refer to the danger situation linked with fear of retaliation as a result of the expression of aggressive impulses; both also recognize that these fears may be coloured by projective mechanisms. The distinction between the two points of view depends therefore not so much on differing concepts as to the mechanism by means of which conflict with reality is handled, but rather on different premises as to the role of external and internal reality in mental development, a matter to which I shall return later.

(3) Hartmann, Kris and Loewenstein (1949) discuss structural conflict involving the ego in a situation where the ego, because of its identification with the object, opposes the completion of aggressive acts. Here, too, we see a statement of general concept which is compatible with some of Melanie Klein's more specific formulations. There is general agreement as to the vagueness of ego boundaries in the early months of life. The close relationship between introjection and identification has been stressed not only by Melanie Klein, but also by Hartmann, Kris and Loewenstein. It is clear, therefore, that the fear of destroying an object with whom the ego is at least partially identified, strongly resembles Melanie Klein's (1935) conception of depressive anxiety, where she described so clearly the infant's anxiety lest his aggressive impulses should result in the destruction of the good internal object. Identification with this object is inevitably closely related to early ego development.

(4) Finally, Hartmann, Kris and Loewenstein refer to structural conflict involving the superego. Here, the incompatibility between their views and those of Melanie Klein does not concern the conceptual description of conflict, but rather the nature and timing of early superego development (again, see Chapter 5). The main point to be emphasized is the compatibility of the conceptual statement with Melanie Klein's views, particularly as it regards the relationship of a severe superego to the continued operation of unmastered aggressive fantasies and impulses.

Since these statements have been taken out of the context of the whole paper, the correlation proposed here should not be taken too literally. True correlation would depend not only on the possible vicissitudes of an instinct, in this instance aggression, but also on other basic assumptions regarding the nature and development of the individual as a whole. Here, for example, there is a basic difference between the two points of view with regard to the relative importance of internal and external reality. For Melanie Klein, internal reality is primary and adaptation to external reality dependent on mastery of the inner world. Hartmann, Kris and Loewenstein, on the other hand, have paid considerable attention to the autonomous development of reality adaptation and would not agree that ego functions depend at every point on a specific mastery of an internal conflict. Anna Freud's position would appear to be intermediate. Melanie Klein pays minimal overt attention to the role of maturation; in contrast, Hartmann, Kris and Loewenstein are very much concerned with this aspect of mental development. Nevertheless, and in spite of these important considerations, it seems that their general formulations regarding the aggressive instinct, like Anna Frued's, are not essentially incompatible with Melanie Klein's point of view.

When, however, an attempt is made to relate Melanie Klein's views on aggression to the nature of the death instinct, more difficult conceptual problems emerge. Freud's (1920) conception of the death instinct, as is well known, was essentially a biological speculation which probably does not belong properly within the field of psychoanalytic theory. According to this view, the death instinct was closely related to the tendency of organic matter to return to an inorganic state of rest. The relation of this tendency to outwardly directed aggressive impulses and even to self-directed destructive impulses of an active nature is highly speculative and controversial. Anna Freud (1949), for example, although she refers to self-destructive behaviour in certain pathological infantile conditions, is careful not to make theoretical hypotheses on this basis. Hartmann, Kris and Loewenstein take a similar position. Melanie Klein, however, has modified Freud's biological conception of the death instinct to put forward a concept of two basic instincts, namely the libido and the death instinct, with the proposal that the death instinct must be considered as an active self-destructive tendency operative from the outset of life. On the basis of this assumption, Melanie Klein has also made the suggestion that anxiety derives from fear of the death instinct, developing from this suggestion far-reaching conclusions both as to the nature of anxiety and as to the meaning or content of early mental conflict. Here, we must consider an interpretation of fundamental analytic concepts of quite a different order from the views of the role of aggression already discussed. With regard to the latter, Melanie Klein is mainly concerned in expanding our knowledge of mental content to include deeper understanding of the role of aggression in early mental life.

It has been shown that many of her propositions regarding early mental conflict and the nature of ambivalence are fully compatible with the general concepts concerning the theory of aggression put forward by Hartmann, Kris and Loewenstein (1949), and also by Anna Freud (1949). Where, however, she expands her own theoretical framework so as to explain her findings on the premise of an active death instinct, it is clear that her work is much more controversial. Here, she has left the field of content elaboration and entered the sphere of conceptual framework. While her elaboration of content, therefore, is not necessarily controversial, her conceptual approach must be regarded as open to question, since she puts forward as fundamental a conception of the death instinct which must itself be regarded as highly speculative and not easily acceptable within the general framework of psychoanalytic thought.

As indicated above, an essential feature of Melanie Klein's work is the emphasis which she places on internal as compared to external reality in the early phases of development. Her views on this question are closely bound up with her premises regarding the basic instincts. The overwhelming importance which she ascribes to inborn destructive impulses, which, in her opinion, exist as an internal threat from the outset of life, combined with her assumption that the destructive impulses follow in their development the libidinal fixation to erotogenic zones, accounts for her preoccupation with the dangers of introjective processes during the early oral phase. This explains the emphasis placed by Melanie Klein and her followers (1952) on the relatively predominant importance of internal reality in early development and the related assumption that introjection and projection are the main, if not only, mental mechanisms in the early months of life. As Hartmann, Kris and Loewenstein (1949) suggest, however, our present state of knowledge does not allow us to accept the proposition that alternating processes of introjection and projection are the only possible explanation of early conflict, nor do they agree that the role of these processes can be solely ascribed to internal forces. Here, they raise the important and long-debated question of the role of external reality and the degree to which aggressive responses can be attributed to frustration rather than to innate destructive tendencies.

> Without discussing the problem whether or not instinctual drives tending toward destructive aims are part of the original equipment of man, one may be satisfied to assume that in the earliest phases of the infant's life any transition from indulgence to deprivation tends to elicit aggressive responses . . . all human relations according to this suggestion may be permanently coloured by the fact that the earliest love relations in the child's life were formed at the time when those whom the child loves are those to whom it owes both indulgence and deprivation (Hartmann *et al.*, 1949).

According to this view, in short, the relation of aggression to external frustration must be taken into account. Anna Freud (1949) approaches the same problem from another point of view. It is her opinion that the existence of innate aggressive tendencies must be accepted. The mastery of these aggressive impulses depends in her view, as in Melanie Klein's (in spite of their somewhat different orientation in other respects), on the fusion of libido with aggression. Failure on the part of the external environment to provide adequate objects for libidinal gratification hampers this task and leads to the appearance of unneutralized aggressive tendencies.

Here, it should be clear, we are in an area where general conceptual thinking must of necessity be somewhat speculative, for the relative importance of object relations is still a matter of controversy. As already indicated, Melanie Klein puts major emphasis on internal factors; external factors are not, however, thereby relegated to a negligible role. Susan Isaacs, for example, in her important paper 'The Nature and Function of Phantasy', explicitly refers to the important role of external frustration as a stimulus for development. She says:

> Disappointment may be the first stimulus to adaptive acceptance of reality, but the postponement of satisfaction and the suspense involved in the complicated learning and thinking about external reality which the child accomplishes . . . can only be endured and sustained when it also satisfies instinctual urges, represented in phantasies, as well. Learning depends upon interest, and interest is derived from desire, curiosity and fear—especially desire and curiosity (1948, p. 108).

This quotation indicates the difference in emphasis of the two approaches. Hartmann, Kris and Loewenstein (1949) clearly indicate that frustration by a loved object is highly significant. Susan Isaacs, dealing with the same problem, stresses the significance of such disappointment in relation to already existing fantasy. In other words, there is an implicit difference between frustration as a *source* of conflict and frustration which will be *interpreted in the light of* inherent conflict and already existing unconscious fantasy. It is the relative importance placed on the latter which distinguishes Melanie Klein and her followers from more orthodox Freudian thought.

It is important to note the close relationship between Melanie Klein's views regarding introjection and projection, her assumptions regarding the nature of the death instinct, and her conceptions of the role of external reality. Since she specifically defines anxiety as a response to the death instinct, it is inevitable that internal danger situations should be regarded as of crucial significance. Since, in addition, she postulates introjection and projection as the main, if not the sole, defensive mechanisms operative in the early months of life, it is relatively easy to understand how far, in her opinion, reality experiences must be influenced by the infant's inner struggles. Moreover, the emphasis given here to a dangerous internal situation as operative from the outset of life explains the importance attached to the progressive internalization of better objects as a crucial feature of early development. Melanie Klein, in referring to internal objects, is concerned essentially with the content of inner fantasy regarding the nature of the inner world. The relationship of these fantasies to the actual environmental situation is implicit rather than explicit. In addition, the emphasis she places on an early differentiation between mechanisms of projection and introjection appears to imply some differentiation between external and internal phenomena from the outset of life. It is therefore difficult to correlate some of her views with basic Freudian concepts concerning the early development of the ego and sense of reality. David Rapaport (1967), for example, has stressed the crucial implications for ego development of the achievement of a differentiation between external and internal reality. He regards the internalization of reality as one of the crucial characteristics of the function of the ego. Heinz Hartmann (1950) also refers to the necessity for the mental apparatus to develop the capacity to recognize internal conflicts. Both of these writers, however, discuss this problem at an abstract level with little or no reference to the explicit fantasies characteristic of the early levels of mental development. The nature of mental conflict in the early months of life remains, of course, a controversial problem. On the one hand, Melanie Klein's emphasis on the internal situation, while at the same time implying sufficient differentiation between internal and external to make a distinction between mechanisms of projection and introjection, does not appear to pay sufficient attention to the role of external reality and the crucial step for ego development implied in the differentiation between external and internal reality. On the other hand, the abstract conceptual approach of Hartmann and Rapaport, while extremely helpful as a frame of reference, may not take into adequate account the possible role of early fantasy life in the development of the infant.

In this connection, it appears that theoretical premises concerning the nature and function of fantasy are crucial. In particular, we touch here on the basic problem of the relation between reality thinking, autonomous functions of the ego, and their unconscious sources. Hartmann (1950), for example, although he indicates very clearly the way in which unconscious fantasy can interfere with secondary process thinking and the reality adaptation of the ego, nevertheless places great importance on the concept of a conflict-free autonomous ego. It would appear implicit in his argument that conflict-free or autonomous ego functions are relatively, if not absolutely, independent of unconscious significance. Susan Isaacs, on the other hand, states:

> In our view reality-thinking cannot operate without concurrent and supporting unconscious phantasies. . . . The fact that phantasy-thinking and reality-thinking have a distinct character when fully developed does not necessarily imply that reality-thinking operates quite independently of unconscious phantasy (1948, p. 108 f.).

This would imply that for Melanie Klein and her followers no mental activity, however functionally free, can be devoid of unconscious significance. Fantasy is, in Isaacs' words, 'the mental expression of instinct'; fantasies therefore play a dominant role in mental life from the outset. According to this point of view, Hartmann's concept of neutralized instinctual energy would appear to be relatively unacceptable. The availability of this energy would appear to depend not primarily on neutralization but rather on the significance of the activity as a gratification of unconscious fantasy. Freedom of activity, in short, would depend on unconscious fantasies which endow the overt activity with unconscious value. It appears that Hartmann's emphasis, by contrast, is on neutralization as a means of liberating instinctual energy from its unconscious sources so that it becomes freely available for the ego.

Here, we appear to be concerned with a genuine difference of opinion as to basic conceptions of the nature of the psychic apparatus. Although extremes of this difference are illustrated here in the contrast between Hartmann and Melanie Klein, the problem may well be crucial for the development of psychoanalytic theory in general. Hartmann's concept, which is correlated with Freud's hints in 'Analysis, Terminable and Interminable' (1937) as to the possibility of inborn ego attributes, stresses the relative unchangeability and autonomy of certain ego functions. Melanie Klein, in contrast, assumes that the unconscious significance of every mental activity may be ultimately traced to instinctual sources and related unconscious fantasies. It is obviously essential, if Melanie Klein's work is to be correlated within the main body of analytic theory, that she should indicate more clearly how true reality testing and secondary process thinking can be understood in terms of her basic premises; how inborn factors affect different phases of mental development; and how maturation plays a role in different stages of development. On the other hand, it appears that, valuable though Hartmann's conception of conflict-free autonomous ego functions may be from a conceptual and descriptive point of view, it is nevertheless desirable that these formulations be correlated more closely with detailed description as to the relationship between neutralization and specific fantasy and conflict.

This correlation of concept and content is significant not only from a theoretical, but from a clinical point of view. The concept of autonomous ego functions relatively divorced from unconscious meaning and possibly arising from innate causes is likely to lead to relative scepticism as to the possibility of effecting major changes in character structure. Under certain circumstances this point of view could possibly encourage an attitude of pessimism and the acceptance of limited therapeutic goals. In contrast, the extreme emphasis placed by Melanie Klein and her followers on the instinctual basis or unconscious significance of all ego attributes with the related tendency to believe that most, if not all, of these attributes should respond to psychoanalysis may, under certain circumstances, encourage over-optimism and difficulty in accepting failure after many years of intensive treatment. Although, as already suggested, the implications of extreme attitudes in either direction are used for purposes of illustration, there are indications that differences in therapeutic approach based on the relative emphasis placed on inborn or autonomous ego features on the one hand, or on unresolved unconscious conflicts on the other, is a vital and open question in psychoanalysis.

In connection with the subject of this chapter, however, we are here concerned not only with the relation of concept to content, but with the influence of basic concepts on problems of clinical application and validation. It is, of course, inevitable that, in the clinical practice of psychoanalysis, theoretical hypotheses influence clinical interpretation. It is, however, extremely important that as clear a distinction as possible should be made between interpretations based on understanding of the content of unconscious conflicts and interpretations based on conceptual hypotheses. Melanie Klein's work, for example, shows very clearly the degree to which conceptual hypotheses may influence interpretation of content. Susan Isaacs' (1948) paper on fantasy illustrates this complicated interrelationship very clearly. In her more general opening remarks concerning the nature and function of fantasy, in her illustrations from the field of general psychology, and in her discussion of Freud's views, she makes contributions to our conceptual framework, which many analysts have found to be valid and significant. As soon, however, as she discusses content, her implicit acceptance of Melanie Klein's concept of the death instinct and her assumption of complex innate knowledge result in propositions regarding the specific content of very early fantasies which many psychoanalysts would find unacceptable.

Close study of the work of those analysts who have given us such valuable contributions towards the reformulation of basic analytic concepts indicates the advantage for such reformulation of considering the individual psychic apparatus in isolation. By this, it is not implied that the need for an object as a means of instinctual gratification is neglected, but that the Freudian concept of primary narcissism and autoerotism is retained as the model of psychic structure in the early days of life. The acceptance of this premise makes possible a consideration of mental development involving a very gradual growth of the ego, the sense of reality, and true object relations. It also facilitates the reformulation of Freud's original views of the psychic apparatus as a means of modifying and controlling instinctual drives.

From many sources, however, we have increasing evidence as to the basic importance of very early object relations. The nature and significance of these early object relationships is still a matter of controversy. It is not impossible that it may prove extremely difficult to conceptualize the meaning of early object relationships in terms of our present theoretical framework. A promising theoretical approach to this problem appears to be implicit in Bertram Lewin's (1950) work on dreams, in which he substitutes for regression to primary narcissism, regression to the most primitive object relationship. The implications of this attempt appear to be far-reaching. Unless some such theoretical hypothesis can be postulated, there is at least the possibility that just as Freud had to abandon his attempt to correlate his psychological findings with the findings of other disciplines, thus making his decisive step in setting up the concept of the mental apparatus, it may become necessary with our increased recognition of the importance of object relationships from the dawn of life to modify our conceptual framework to take fully into account the object needs of the human infant. Inevitably we will also be faced in this connection with an evaluation of the psychological significance of these early objective experiences with the possibility that Susan Isaacs' approach to the nature and function of fantasy may prove to be of outstanding importance. It may, in short, be inadequate to retain a concept of primary narcissism and to include therein the lack of differentiation of infant and mother in the early days of life. Much as this might be desirable from the point of view of coherent theoretical formulation, it may indeed prove that psychoanalytic truth cannot be adequately expressed in abstract conceptual terms based on the individual psychic apparatus. Here, finally, we may be concerned with an insuperable limitation of the conceptual approach. This suggestion, however, may be premature at this point since, in the first place, we have by no means exhausted the possibilities of conceptual reformulation and, in the second place, the role of object relations in early infancy still remains open to debate.

An allied, but somewhat different, difficulty in the formulation of abstract concepts concerns the nature and function of the superego. Although there are many difficulties inherent in the conceptual reformulation of Freudian theory, using Freud's model of the mental apparatus as the basis for detailed consideration of ego structure, these difficulties do not appear to be insuperable, as David Rapaport (1967) so clearly indicates. With regard to the superego, however, it seems that conceptual reformulation has, up to now, raised a number of difficulties, some intimately related to the present stage of theoretical knowledge. The attention paid by most analysts to superego structure and function in the early period of a structural approach has, to a very considerable extent, now been overshadowed by the emphasis on the ego and its defences. While the latter lends itself fairly readily to reformulation in abstract conceptual terms related to Freud's original conception of the mental apparatus, the superego is less easy to formulate in abstract conceptual terms. Edward Glover, referring to the same problem, states: 'The superego concept is from first to last a clinical concept. It was founded on clinical analysis, and retains throughout a clinical connotation. One must distinguish carefully between descriptions of the superego and theories of its origins' (1947, p. 489). This, too, is clearly indicated in the Hartmann, Kris and Loewenstein paper 'Comments on the Formation of Psychic Structure' (1946). Although their formulation of the earlier period and of the development of ego functions remains fundamentally abstract and conceptual, their description of superego formation is formulated in terms of a specific meaningful situation, i.e. the oedipal conflict. Here, in short, it has not been possible clearly to separate concept from content up to the present time. A full discussion of the reason for, or nature of, this problem would involve detailed discussion of controversial views regarding the origin of the superego, which would be outside the scope of this chapter. The point is raised mainly to indicate the extreme difficulty of separating content from concept in relation to certain aspects of analytic theory.

While, therefore, there can be no doubt as to the extreme importance of as objective a formulation as possible of our fundamental concepts, I have tried to indicate some of the possible obstacles to achievement. The essentially concrete subjective nature of the material with which we are dealing leads to real difficulties in clear separation of theory from practice. This chapter, however, is not primarily concerned with this basic problem. Our theory, according to this point of view, must be concerned not only with abstract formulations, but with interpretations of meaningful content, sufficiently general to be included under the heading of theory, rather than described as specific clinical observations. The analyst, for example, is definitely basing his deductions on a theoretical hypothesis of this nature when he interprets certain symbols, oedipal fantasies and well-accepted conflicts of the pregenital period. Both increased depth and wider applications of our knowledge lead to new findings with regard to content which, however valuable they may prove as a source of stimulation and the opening of new vistas into the unconscious mind, must be correlated with the general body of analytic knowledge. In addition, however, to this aspect of psychoanalytic theory, the search instigated by Freud (1900) in 'The Interpretation of Dreams' for an abstract conceptual framework has been continued up to the present, as illustrated in this chapter by reference to the recent work of Hartmann, Kris, Loewenstein and Rapaport. It is essential for the progress of our knowledge that, on the one hand, expansions of our theory mainly concerned with content should be correlated within this general conceptual framework. Equally important is the need for abstract conceptual formulations to be related to interpretations of content. This need of mutual correlation is of importance not only in respect of our general body of theoretical knowledge, but also in respect of important clinical implications. The contributions of Melanie Klein, used as a basis for illustration in this chapter, clearly show the disadvantage of inadequate distinction between content and concept. It is unfortunate that this confusion has inevitably led to relative neglect of many of her valuable contributions in the sphere of content (see Chapter 5).

8

THE DOCTOR–PATIENT RELATIONSHIP IN PSYCHIATRY[1]

(1966)

In this chapter I will attempt to bring together some of the considerations relevant to the relationship between psychiatry and psychoanalysis which have been either explicit or implicit in preceding chapters. Since, in addition, a discussion of psychotherapy inevitably involves some consideration of the differences between various forms of psychotherapy and traditional psychoanalysis, some reference will be made to questions which are considered in greater detail in the second section of this volume.

The preceding chapters in this section were not based primarily on the clinical practice of psychoanalysis. Rather, the most common symptoms of patients seeking psychiatric help, namely anxiety and depression, have been considered in terms of their developmental significance. The capacity to recognize, tolerate and master both of these basic affects has been related to the evaluation of patients seen in a wide variety of clinical situations. As regards anxiety, a differentiation has been made between primitive forms of externally-directed separation anxiety and the more mature, potentially challenging anxiety which arises as a signal of internal danger. In the case of depression, a similar distinction has been drawn between the depression which is appropriate to certain situations of developmental or situational stress or loss and the depression which bears evidence to developmental failure. In the preceding chapter the importance of object relations in the early development of the individual child was emphasized. In this chapter I hope to expand this last point, which I believe is highly relevant to the doctor–patient relationship in psychiatric evaluation and psychiatric treatment.

[1] Adapted from a paper entitled 'Transference in Psychotherapy', which was presented at a Symposium on the Role of Transference in Psychotherapy held on 20 May 1966 at the Department of Psychiatry, Tufts University School of Medicine.

Both evaluation and treatment, whatever its nature, take place in the setting of a one-to-one relationship. It is a major thesis of this chapter that both the quality and the stability of this relationship provide invaluable evidence of the level of development which the patient can achieve. Although it does not duplicate the original developmental process, the doctor–patient relationship does nevertheless draw on strengths and reveal weaknesses of certain fundamental attributes acquired early in life. No one, moreover, is so mature or stable that these attributes may not be undermined under conditions of specific stress. Some of these, as will be discussed presently, may be concomitant to the therapeutic situation. Since it has long been recognized that a limited regressive process is an integral feature of the transference neurosis in psychoanalysis, a major goal of this chapter is to differentiate between the type of regression which may ultimately further mastery and adaptation and the forms of repression which undermine previously available basic ego attributes.

In recent years psychiatry and related disciplines have been increasingly confronted by the magnitude of the demands on their services. New techniques have been introduced in the hope that they may deal effectively with psychological problems which cannot be met by offering long-term individual treatment and/or guidance or casework to all of the patients who seek psychological help. Short-term treatment (i.e. time-limited treatment with techniques directed towards specific, limited goals) has become increasingly popular in many psychiatric clinics. Group therapy and family therapy have found a justified place among our technical procedures. Careful and appropriate use of the rapidly expanding pharmacological products has an important place in the rehabilitation of many individuals who might otherwise require prolonged hospitalization. Community psychiatry, which includes prophylactic measures and various methods of indirect intervention, has come to the forefront of many psychiatric departments, associations and training programmes.

Some of these measures, like the development of group therapy, prophylactic selection procedures and time-limited therapy during the years of World War II, were originally stimulated by the demands of expediency. Their subsequent growth and recent revival suggest, however, that they may in certain cases prove not only more practicable, but sometimes more effective than intensive individual therapy in an open-ended treatment situation. In so far, therefore, as psychoanalysis is to be regarded as a comprehensive discipline, the success or failure of different therapeutic approaches should be formulated in relation to the landmarks of individual psychological development. Such understanding may, first, prove the value of a psychoanalytic approach in the initial evaluation of the psychiatric patient. It should, second, help in the selection of the most appropriate treatment for individual patients. It should, finally, enable us to differentiate between success or failure mainly determined by the patient's assets or liabilities, and results largely attributable to the fact that the therapist has failed either in his personal interaction with the patient or in his choice of the technique which might best have served his patient's needs.

In this chapter it will be necessary to review the principal features of one-to-one relationships. In so doing, my main purpose is to pinpoint those aspects of the doctor–patient relationship which determine a satisfactory therapeutic situation. The realistic factors of this relationship must therefore be distinguished as far as possible from distortions, fears and unrealistic expectations. Consideration of the latter involves differentiation between distortions attributable to a reversible decompensation in the patient, distortions attributable to defects in the psychiatrist's technique, and those distortions which reflect such serious or irreversible problems in the patient that a question should be raised as to what psychotherapeutic goals may justifiably be anticipated.

I have already suggested that certain crucial aspects of definitive psychic structure and function are initiated in the setting of the original one-to-one parent–child relationship. These attributes are normally subject to some regressive impairment and subsequent reintegration during later developmental crises (see Chapter 16). Unless, however, they have been successfully initiated during the earliest years, serious questions must be raised as to how far psychotherapy, either during adolescence or in adult life, can help the seriously handicapped individual to acquire psychological capacities which had not been initiated at the age-appropriate time. Unless, in other words, the in-individual possesses some capacity to internalize and identify, and to recognize and tolerate some affective pain, and in addition is genuinely motivated to respond adaptively to developmental challenges, too much cannot be anticipated regarding his or her potential to become genuinely autonomous.

Individuals suffering from serious developmental defects are not only handicapped in their capacity for emotional growth; they are also particularly vulnerable to regressive responses to developmental and situational stress. In predisposed individuals such regressive responses may result in the relatively irreversible impairment which characterizes the typical forms of psychotic illness. Here the psychiatrist will know within a relatively brief period of time that he is confronted by an extremely difficult, if not impossible, therapeutic problem. Attempts to form relationships with very disturbed psychotics are to be regarded as important and challenging learning experiences during the training of psychiatrists. Such patients provide invaluable first-hand evidence of the distortions, magical thinking and omnipotent fantasies which impair their one-to-one relations. Many of these patients cannot achieve or maintain a sufficiently confident relationship gradually to relinquish magical expectations or to accept some of the limitations of reality. These goals may sometimes be partially achieved. For this to occur, however, a long-term investment, often indefinitely extended, is necessary. Such treatment obviously cannot be provided for the large majority of psychotic hospitalized patients. It should be recognized, moreover, that drug treatment, the provision of adequate structure, family therapy and group therapy are all measures which are compatible with a developmental understanding of the patient's definitive deficits. Such measures may help substantially in bringing about clinical improvement, e.g. remission or rehabilitation. They may also militate against the emergence of the extremely intense, possibly unmanageable, therapeutic situation which may develop if and when the treatment of such patients is limited to an exclusive one-to-one relationship.

Both developmental failure and a relatively irreversible regressive process characterize the familiar subgroups of clinical schizophrenia, which may of course be at least partially determined by genetic factors. Such factors must also be acknowledged in respect of manic depressive illness. A crucial and not sufficiently recognized diagnostic problem relates to the differentiation between psychotic patients and individuals subject to reversible regressive processes during periods of maturational or situational stress. These patients, who belong to the groups usually described as borderline, schizo-affective characters or primitive hysterics, typically suffer from some developmental failure in the area of early one-to-one relationships. They are, in addition, particularly vulnerable to substantial regression in respect of prolonged or excessive stress. This may undermine previously available ego functions, including the capacity to distinguish between fantasy and reality. In contrast to the psychotic, however, such regression is often transient and totally reversible. These individuals subsequently prove capable of establishing a one-to-one relationship which helps them to remobilize their previous achievements. Such relationships, for reasons which will be elaborated presently, should, however, be limited in respect of both their goals and their intensity. As noted in Chapter 6, the therapy indicated for patients of this type involves consolidation and reintegration of earlier achievements in the setting of a stable relationship.

In some cases this therapeutic relationship is the first real relationship which the patient has ever established. This, in combination with the earlier developmental failure, may make it difficult if not impossible to reach a definitive termination. The patient's capacity to achieve and maintain a genuine object relationship has improved. The capacity to internalize and subsequently to achieve genuine autonomy may, however, remain substantially limited. In my own experience a number of patients falling into this group have been able to maintain a high degree of both personal and professional adaptation, providing the psychiatrist remains available for occasional interviews or consultation. This type of extended, though non-intensive, therapy is often devalued as merely supportive. It may be suggested, however, that an arrangement based on mutual acknowledgement of the patient's limitations in a specific area is in the first place in keeping with psychoanalysis as a comprehensive developmental psychology. It comprises in addition a form of treatment which, at relatively little expense, time or effort, can often maintain a high degree of adaptation in individuals who might otherwise become serious psychiatric casualties.

Both the initial evaluation and the most effective treatment of patients falling into this category, however, present a number of problems. As already indicated, a reversible regression may initially be diagnosed as a schizophrenic illness. An example of this not infrequent diagnostic error was cited in Chapter 1. In such cases it should be relatively easy for the evaluating psychiatrist to reach the conclusion that the patient's vulnerability to regression was suggestive of serious developmental failure. Such patients, in brief, like those described as so-called good hysterics (see Chapter 14), have not acquired the basic ego attributes which facilitate a stable doctor–patient relationship. Although the manifest content of their verbalized fantasy may, as in that case, appear to be both genital and oedipal, this symptomatic façade is highly deceptive. When, as in the case described, such patients have regressed sufficiently to raise a question as to whether or not they may not be psychotic, the psychiatrist will be alerted to the possible risks integral to any attempt at prolonged or intensive psychotherapy.

Unfortunately, however, a particular hazard in the evaluation of many patients suffering from serious developmental failure is attributable to the fact that they may first seek psychiatric help regarding symptoms which clearly appear to be mainly neurotic, i.e. obsessional or hysterical. In such cases the psychoanalytically orientated psychiatrist may be tempted to make a diagnosis based on the level of instinctual fixation or regression reflected in the patient's manifest symptomatology. Over the past thirty years I have seen or have been consulted about well over a hundred patients who suffered to a greater or lesser degree from this type of developmental failure. At best, there are the patients who, if first seen during a period of developmental or situational stress, can respond effectively to a structured time-limited period of therapy. Recent experience with such treatment, conducted by psychiatric residents during their last year of training, has demonstrated, first, that a time-limited treatment may be prophylactic against the emergence of a regressive, highly dependent therapeutic situation. It has also indicated the degree to which regression during stressful periods may be as deceptive as the manifest neurotic symptomatology of patients suffering from serious developmental failure. In other words, decompensated but nevertheless potentially mature individuals can integrate within a relatively brief period of time a new and stable ego identification. Such treatment illustrates in addition the positive value, whether or not major conflicts have been definitively resolved, of careful and sensitive handling of the process of separation, i.e. termination. Such treatment, in brief, is not directed towards the emergence and interpretation of regressive transference fantasies. It is focused, first, towards the establishment of a good doctor–patient relationship; second, towards the patient's utilization of this relationship through a process of progressive internalization; and third, towards facilitating the definitive integration of this internalization in the service of the patient's autonomy and independence.

Unfortunately, however, these goals are not always easy to achieve. As already noted, certain patients do not appear to be capable of achieving the final therapeutic goal. In other words, they cannot work through a genuine separation and termination. Moreover, it is not always possible to predict at the time of initial evaluation every patient's capacity for emotional growth. On the one hand, certain patients in my own experience, both as a therapist and as a teacher, have done far better than was originally anticipated. In retrospect it has become evident that these patients had been decompensated at the time of psychiatric evaluation. When such decompensation has resulted mainly in overt depression, the patient's initial description of his own premorbid personality and achievements has been distorted as a result of his diminished self-esteem. One such patient is briefly described in Chapter 6.

Conversely, however, some patients have done less well than had been initially anticipated. The majority of such patients had been evaluated during late adolescence or early adult life. A number of them had been diagnosed as analysable neurotics. Their subsequent regression during analysis or closely related techniques of psychotherapy has clearly revealed the dangers of this type of diagnostic error. Understanding of both the successes and the failures requires careful differentiation between the real doctor–patient relationship, distortions in this relationship attributable to developmental failure, and finally, the role of transference in psychotherapy. It is my conviction that many problems encountered in the conduct of psychotherapy arise from confusion between certain repetitive elements inevitably reflected in all one-to-one relationships, i.e. transference in its most generalized meaning, and the emergence of transference fantasies as a specific constellation during the course of treatment.

'In order to effect a cure a condition of expectant faith has been recognized for centuries as an essential prerequisite.' This statement, written sixty years ago by Sigmund Freud, remains as relevant today as it was at the time when it was written. I have so far emphasized the fact that the doctor–patient relationship is first and foremost a one-to-one relationship. Freud's statement described in ordinary language the non-verbal affective attitude towards a trusted person which characterizes a good doctor–patient relationship. It is thus a cardinal feature of all individual psychotherapy in which doctor and patient achieve what may be described as a good therapeutic alliance. It must be recognized, however, that few patients, whatever their ultimate diagnosis, can establish such a relationship without appropriate efforts on the part of the psychiatrist.

Most successful doctors, in whatever speciality, acknowledge and attempt to alleviate their patient's initial anxieties and distortions. This is a prerequisite for the establishment of a confident doctor–patient relationship and clearly influences the patient's subsequent response to any form of treatment. When such treatment is physical and specific, it may be relatively easy to separate those therapeutic factors which result from the human doctor–patient relationship from those attributable to specific measures recommended for the patient's presenting problem. In psychiatry, however, the very difficulties which have led the patient to seek help are inevitably reflected in his initial responses. This makes it both more difficult and more important to make a conceptual and clinical differentiation between the real doctor–patient relationship, distortions attributable to the patient's relative incapacity to form such a relationship, and finally, the emergence of specific transference material. I am thus raising a question as to how far every affective attitude which interferes with the patient's perception of his therapist as a real person is attributable to a regressive transference reaction.

Every patient referred to a psychiatrist will bring to his first interview affective responses or the defences against them which reflect both his general and his immediate capacity for confident object relations. All patients have some residual vulnerabilities which influence their responses to each new relationship. Many psychiatrists and psychoanalysts tend to regard the resultant affect or distortions as evidence of a genuine transference reaction. Is this, however, actually the case? For example, if a patient who has always been fearful of authority figures demonstrates anxiety during his initial psychiatric interview, is this response to be regarded as evidence of transference in its traditional meaning? May it not rather derive from a personality attribute which conforms to David Rapaport's definition of psychic structure as 'that part of the psychic apparatus which is only capable of slow and gradual change'? In the most general sense the patient transfers to the therapist his characteristic mode of reacting to one-to-one relationships. This reaction is not, however, to be regarded as a response to the actual personality or technique of the previously unknown psychiatrist. The psychiatrist who acknowledges this type of initial response is not therefore making a transference interpretation. He is rather helping the patient to recognize some of the barriers which might otherwise interfere with the establishment of a good therapeutic alliance.

An additional problem derives from the fact that many patients who seek psychotherapy are first seen at a time when their optimal capacities have already been somewhat impaired by anxiety, depression or a wide variety of neurotic symptoms. Since these, like a transference neurosis, are attributable to a partial regressive process it is hardly surprising that many patients, while waiting for their first interview, develop anticipatory fantasies and wishes which at first sight closely resemble a transference neurosis. Such fantasies are partly attributable to the regressive emergence of the patient's unrealistic hopes and fears. They are sometimes compounded by the patient's preconception of the psychiatrist as someone endowed with almost magical power. They are not in any way determined by the personality of the as yet unseen psychiatrist but derive almost exclusively from the patient's fantasies about psychiatry and psychotherapy. Such pre-treatment fantasies will obviously influence the patient's initial response to the individual psychiatrist as a real person. Unless and until they are counterbalanced by a genuine reaction to the psychiatrist as an individual, a premature and specious transference may be displaced on to the person of the therapist. In brief, the regressive processes already discussed may interfere with the establishment of what Freud described as expectant faith during the initial phases of treatment.

These problems are compounded by a situation more common in the practice of psychiatry than in other forms of medical treatment. Many patients first seen by a consultant are referred to a junior colleague on the explicit understanding that psychotherapy will be undertaken. It is all too common that a relatively young psychiatrist will tend to regard himself as committed in advance to treating a patient on the basis of a relatively brief verbal or written report. His sometimes unjustified faith in the diagnostic skill of a senior colleague may in addition undermine his confidence in his own evaluation of the patient's assets, liabilities and motivation for treatment. Treatment may thus begin at the first meeting without any preliminary period of evaluation or the formulation of explicit, mutually acceptable therapeutic plans and goals. Conversely, it is equally common that patients thus referred begin psychotherapy as passive, rather helpless recipients of a single definitive referral. They may not feel any sense of autonomy or freedom of choice in the event that their emotional responses to the therapist in question are strongly negative from the outset. When, for example, a therapist's appearance, personality traits and mannerisms are forcibly reminiscent of an important person in respect of the patient's unresolved conflicts, such factors may substantially interfere with the establishment of a genuine doctor–patient relationship.

When in these complex situations a psychiatrist acknowledges, and if necessary expresses, his patient's anxieties or unreal expectations, such interventions are not to be regarded as transference interpretations. They might be described rather as clarification of pre-treatment pseudo-transference fantasies which might otherwise interfere with the establishment of a genuine relationship. Similar considerations may also be raised regarding the therapist's approach to infantile demanding patients who express from the outset exaggerated dependence and an attitude which conveys their tendency to seek in the therapist someone endowed with omnipotent powers. If, therefore, the psychiatrist conveys his desire to help, his wish to enlist the patient's active co-operation, and warns the patient against the pain which will result if he persists in unrealistic hopes, such interventions are to be regarded as serious efforts to communicate with the patient at his most mature level, acknowledging but not fostering his unrealistic hopes.

I am thus suggesting that not all distortions which interfere with the patient's initial perception of the psychiatrist are attributable to transference in its traditional meaning. Such distortions may be determined by relatively stable aspects of the patient's capacity to achieve and maintain a genuine and constant object relationship. Although transference in its most general meaning may be recognized, these responses are more attributable to the patient's psychic structure (ego and superego) than to the regressive emergence of previously unconscious fantasies and wishes. When, however, a patient has sought treatment as a result of regressive impairment there is a strong probability that pre-treatment fantasies will also influence the patient's initial perception of the psychiatrist. Early clarification of anxiety, suspicion, unrealistic hopes and dependent longings, whatever their origin, are not, in my opinion, to be regarded as transference interpretations. In such interventions the psychiatrist is attempting to elicit and to reinforce the patient's optimal capacity to establish a meaningful doctor–patient relationship.

I have already indicated that many patients, while waiting for their first psychiatric interview, develop anticipatory fantasies and wishes which closely resemble a transference neurosis. In so far as these fantasies are immediately attached to the person of the therapist, pre-transference fantasies may soon be compounded and intensified by further transference repression. Whether or not this occurs depends on two major factors. First, how far the therapist has been able to take appropriate steps to mobilize the patient's sense of reality, thus removing certain reversible distortions; second, how far the patient is genuinely capable of achieving and maintaining a stable one-to-one relationship.

It is necessary in this context to make a distinction between interpretation of the unconscious meaning of pre-transference fantasies and appropriate responses to the patient's presenting affect. Although the therapist may be presented with considerable evidence as to the specific content of such pre-treatment fantasies, particularly in the treatment of primitive or so-called hysterics, it is seldom, if ever, advisable to make explicit transference interpretations. In so far as these patients are not capable of making a meaningful distinction between transference and reality, interpretation is often experienced as seductive, thus inviting an intense and demanding response on the part of the patient.

It is nevertheless essential that the therapist should respond to the patient's presenting affect and initial reactions to the doctor–patient relationship. Failures in this specific area not only during evaluation but at every stage of treatment may be seriously conducive to regression in the patient. When a psychiatrist can be seen by the patient, but is not heard, and at the same time maintains an expression which reveals no affective response, the therapeutic situation and the transference which emerges may be more regressive in respect of the patient's ego functions than the anticipated but limited regression which is a common and understood feature of the analytic situation.

The doctor–patient relationship has reality features equally important in all forms of treatment. Premature transference interpretation, as already indicated, not only increases the likelihood of a transference regression; it also interferes with the initiation of a genuine doctor–patient relationship. Silence and detachment may have very much the same effect. Acknowledgement of the patient's immediate feelings, particularly those which result in affective distortion, will, in contrast, further the establishment of a viable therapeutic situation.

There are wide variations in our patient population as to the degree to which they are, or have previously been, capable of maintaining stable one-to-one object relations. I have already noted the diagnostic difficulties presented by patients whose manifest symptomatology appears to be hysterical. In such cases the therapist's previous commitment to the patient or the patient's excessive attachment to a therapist endowed with omnipotent powers may become a serious additional handicap. In this context, the more the patient insists that there is only one therapist with whom he can work, the more difficult it may become to manage a highly regressive transference situation. When, in these circumstances, a therapist responds by regarding such material as an indication for increased interpretative activity, more frequent appointments and telephone calls, an already difficult situation may become virtually impossible.

Over the course of many years as a supervisor and consultant I have seen more patients than I can count who had been allowed to remain in such regressive situations. A vicious circle has developed, determined on the one hand by the patient's intense transference and lack of therapeutic alliance, and on the other by the therapist's commitment, frustration and countertransference reactions. This has resulted in increasing decompensation of the patient's autonomous ego functions. Many of these patients have ended in hospital. In a number, however, their responses to an approach directed towards remobilization of their previous achievements has shown that the regression had been unnecessary and harmful. Sometimes both patient and therapist had been involved in a regressive situation which could not be broken without outside intervention. This unfortunate development can often be avoided by early recognition of the patient's tendency to develop this type of negative therapeutic reaction.

Such patients, it may be suggested, have frequently failed to reach a level of development at which they could establish a confident, trusting one-to-one relationship. Fortunately, however, not all of our patients suffer from such serious handicaps. Though vulnerable, they may be potentially capable of establishing a real doctor–patient relationship. They may also possess the capacity to integrate a positive ego identification. As a rule these patients have also previously experienced a triangular conflict. Pre-treatment transference fantasies, however, will not prevent the more mature neurotic patient from establishing a real doctor–patient relationship. As treatment continues, such patients may later report dream and fantasy material which suggests the emergence of a genuine transference neurosis.

The specific content of the transference neurosis will, for these more mature patients, be considerably influenced by the respective sexes of patient and therapist. Successful resolution of the infantile neurosis implies that the child has succeeded in retaining good object relations with both parents. The child will, on the whole, tend to identify with the parent of the same sex. The child likes, and wishes to be liked more by, the parent of the other sex. Few of our patients, whether analytic or therapeutic, have achieved an ideal resolution of this triangular conflict. In classical analysis the transference neurosis involves revival and interpretation of all aspects of the triangle. Just how far is this goal appropriate to the conduct of other forms of therapy? Some of our patients are, as has been suggested, incapable of experiencing a triangular conflict. For others (particularly patients during developmental crises) it may be both unnecessary and undesirable to encourage the emergence of a sexual or hostile regressive transference neurosis.

Let us take the not atypical case of a relatively young woman who, despite many strengths, is unable to establish a satisfactory heterosexual relationship. Her difficulties may be predominantly attributable to her lack of a sense of secure feminine identity. In traditional psychoanalysis the resolution of this problem would involve the revival of her incestuous fantasies, at the same time increasing hostile rivalry with her mother. In therapy with a woman, this girl might develop not only a positive therapeutic alliance, but also a positive identification with her therapist. This identification might arise as the result of positive transference, which then decreased her capacity to deal effectively with previously unresolved ambivalence towards her own mother. This could raise her self-esteem, diminish the harshness of her superego and enable her to internalize a better and more feminine ego-ideal.

In some cases a lasting improvement may result from just this type of positive transference identification. It is my impression that such results are impeded rather than helped by explicit verbal interpretation. Both patient and therapist nevertheless implicitly acknowledge the source of the patient's symptomatic improvement. It is important that the therapist who succeeds in this way should not feel dissatisfied by the result of his treatment. He should not, in short, confront himself with the analytic ideal of mastery as a result of transference interpretation and depreciate the value of mastery or insight through progressive use of transference identification. Such patients often profit by a relatively short course of psychotherapy, after which they usually need a period of interruption during which they may consolidate their gains. In some cases no further help may be asked for or indicated. Other patients (e.g. adolescents who have successfully utilized this type of therapy) may return after a time as adults who recognize internal conflict, rather than as adolescents still in need of objects for identification. These may then prove to be patients for whom traditional psychoanalysis becomes the treatment of choice.

The same young woman, it may be suggested, might achieve an equally satisfactory result with a male therapist who, by implicitly acknowledging her feminine traits, could help her then to identify herself with his perception of her as a woman. The gratification implicit in this type of transference reaction is not necessarily to be regarded as primitive or incestuous, i.e. regressive. It is rather comparable with the successful aim-inhibited relationship achieved in a successful post-oedipal father–daughter relationship. As suggested earlier, explicit interpretation of the primitive incestuous wishes towards the father or of the hostile rivalry which precedes a secure identification with the mother will seldom further this type of transference response. Unless and until it has been definitely decided that psychoanalysis, or its closest equivalent, is indicated and necessary for a progressive result, transference interpretation is not likely to help. In most cases of the sort we are discussing, it will increase the probability of regression. While some transference manifestations are almost inevitable, it is seldom desirable, at least in the initial stages of psychotherapy, to foster their expression. In so far as transference interpretation is both indicated and successful, I believe we are in reality discussing a modified psychoanalysis rather than psychotherapeutic treatment using other techniques.

This conclusion might be amplified as follows. In traditional psychoanalysis the transference is interpreted, while the real object relationship is often so secure that it seldom needs explicit reinforcement. The therapist's efforts are directed towards helping the patient to achieve the genuine conviction as to his primitive psychic reality which, when analysis is definitely indicated, is a necessary preliminary to genuine mastery. In most therapy, in contrast, while transference may be obvious to the therapist, it is the reality of the relationship which remains in the forefront. It is the strengthening of the real object relationship which holds the potential for considerably increasing the patient's insight. This insight, however, is frequently utilized by the patient in his relationships outside the therapeutic situation. In some young persons the adolescent re-emergence of specific unresolved conflicts makes further transference regression redundant, since mastery and adaptation are so near to integration.

A problematic therapeutic situation arises when patients who were originally seen during a period of serious decompensation improve during the course of successful psychotherapy and become, as a result, capable of developing a genuine transference neurosis. In such an eventuality, new decisions become necessary. Should the therapist, if qualified, change his technique to that of traditional psychoanalysis? If not, should treatment be interrupted, with the possible plan of subsequent referral for psychoanalysis? Should the transference be utilized without attempting explicit interpretations? Finally, when should the therapist decide to make the transference neurosis in its difficulty and complexity the central focus of treatment? Such decisions can only be made in context and by the individual therapist. It remains, however, prerequisite that the patient remains capable of maintaining the real doctor–patient relationship as the transference develops. As already suggested, in those patients in whom a partial and substitute gratification or transference identification with the therapist is enhancing the patient's capacity for genuine emotional growth, interpretation of its unconscious meaning is not only unnecessary; it may indeed prove a deterrent rather than an aid to progress.

The doctor–patient relationship is crucial in forming the setting in which therapy is initiated and continued, or when therapy becomes almost indistinguishable from traditional psychoanalysis. It is no less important during the period of termination. Unless the therapy has fostered a regressive situation, it is to be expected that most patients will show progressive movement. Transference regression during the later stages of treatment is one indication for introducing the possibility of termination. In many cases termination may be suggested by the patient's increasing wishes for greater autonomy and independence. Its determination and implementation should never be decided unilaterally by either patient or therapist. Just as the initiation of treatment should be a mutual decision, so should its termination be.

In this context it is also desirable that both patient and therapist should agree that the patient feel free to return. The error of ascribing transference meaning to distortions in fact determined by ego characteristics is, unfortunately, often repeated during the closing phases of all forms of psychotherapy. For those patients who suffer from ego defects, the therapist may have been the first person with whom he had achieved a genuine relationship. To ascribe his anxiety about impending termination entirely to regressive transference expressions is to minimize the importance of the real relationship. As already noted, certain patients in this category are so handicapped in their capacity to achieve and maintain a positive ego identification that some contact (often quite infrequent and irregular) must be continued indefinitely. These patients are in essence to be regarded as relatively interminable.

In conclusion, I have attempted first to consider the relevance of the doctor–patient relationship to the evaluation of typical presenting differences between psychotics, non-psychotic patients suffering from either serious developmental failure or reversible regressive states, and potentially healthy neurotic adults. The last two groups comprise a major proportion of patients referred to a psychiatrist for psychotherapy. I have therefore focused primarily on the significance of the real doctor–patient relationship, first, during the period of initial evaluation; second, during the course of treatment; and last, but by no means least, as the central feature of the process of termination. I have suggested, in summary, the dangers of attributing every distortion in this relationship to transference in its traditional meaning. I have indicated the need to differentiate between distortions attributable to relatively stable aspects of the patient's definitive psychic structure and function, those attributable to regression precipitated by specific stress, those which indicate the emergence of pre-treatment pseudo-transference fantasies, and finally, those which suggest the emergence of a classical transference neurosis during the course of treatment. Whatever technique may be chosen as appropriate during the process of psychotherapy, the fact that individual psychotherapy involves a one-to-one dyadic relationship cannot be over-emphasized. The establishment of such a relationship will draw on the strengths and reveal the vulnerabilities acquired during the original developmental process. It is the task of the therapist to elicit during treatment the optimal capacities of the patient as a foundation without which no therapeutic technique can be effective.

Section II

Clinical Psychoanalysis

9

INTRODUCTION

During my last years in London I had my first formal opportunity to apply general psychiatric experience to a specific psychoanalytic goal, namely the selection of patients for supervised analysis by candidates in training. As Assistant Director of the London Clinic of Psychoanalysis, I shared with the Director the responsibility of evaluating patients who applied to the Clinic for psychoanalytic treatment. This proved to be a stimulating but somewhat frustrating task. Many of the patients seen for evaluation were reminiscent of a statement made by Freud:

> I have been able to elaborate and to test my therapeutic method only on severe, indeed on the severest cases. . . . Psycho-analytic therapy was created through and for the treatment of patients permanently unfit for existence, and its triumph has been that it has made a satisfactorily large number of these permanently *fit* for existence (1905*a*, p. 263).

This situation reflected the relative lack of integration and communication between psychoanalysis and organized psychiatry in England. Few if any patients seen at evaluative interviews appear retrospectively to have met what I now consider to be the major criteria for analysability. Most of the patients came on their own initiative, often for somewhat doubtful reasons. The majority of those referred by psychiatrists or other clinics were mainly sent as a last resort. Before leaving London in 1949 I had ample opportunity to confirm my impression that overt neurotic symptomatology, whether hysterical or obsessional, could not be regarded as conclusive evidence that a patient was suffering from an analysable neurotic disorder. Such symptomatology, it soon became clear, was not inconsistent with serious psychopathology and subsequent failure to develop an analysable transference neurosis.

One of the first patients I interviewed, for example, was a disarming, apparently highly motivated young man suffering from disabling obsessional symptoms. This patient, previously a conscientious objector, had developed incapacitating symptoms following a relatively severe head injury. I came to the conclusion that he was too disturbed to be suitable for analysis by a candidate in training. I found him, however, sufficiently interesting to accept him as my own clinic patient. The degree of his disability was similar to that described by Freud (1905*a*). The initial favourable impression he created was, however, comparable to Freud's description of the obsessional patient whose analysis proved to be therapeutically successful (1909*a*; see also Chapter 13).

The early phases of this patient's analysis have been discussed elsewhere (Rosenberg, 1946). The outcome of his treatment is, however, relevant to this second section, which is predominantly concerned with clinical psychoanalysis. After a relatively brief period in which he developed an intense, over-idealized positive transference, his underlying hostility towards women led to the emergence of an intensely negative reaction. The underlying helpless rage against his mother emerged increasingly in the analytic situation. Certain paranoid tendencies which had been noted from the outset became increasingly evident as time went on. Treatment was interrupted by mutual agreement after approximately one year.

At the time I was mainly interested in direct confrontation of the rage and hostility which often underlie conscious expressions of fanatical pacifism. It was at the same time disturbing to recognize and to acknowledge the degree to which this patient's apparent motivation and initial positive responses had been deceptive. The reaction formations which had determined his initial passive compliance were certainly different from those which Freud described in the history of the Rat Man (1909*a*). They had been initiated at a far more primitive level, deriving in essence from failure to resolve ambivalence in the early mother–child relationship. He was thus unable to establish a genuine therapeutic alliance before unavoidable reality factors increased his regressive transference to a degree which impaired his perception of reality.

It was possible for me to resume the evaluation of patients applying for supervised analysis soon after my transfer to the Boston Institute. For more than fifteen years I served either as Chairman or Consultant to the Committee responsible for the selection of such patients. The initial findings of our group have been reported elsewhere (see Knapp *et al.*, 1960). Briefly to summarize our first report: Of the first hundred patients interviewed, none of those accepted had an obsessional neurosis of a severity comparable to that of the patient described above. The majority of patients accepted with a diagnosis of obsessional neurosis or obsessional character were relatively well-defended individuals who presented no undue difficulties in the establishment of an analytic situation. Relatively few of them, however, had developed an overt analysable transference neurosis during the first year of analytic treatment. This finding suggests that our interviewers were in general alert to the relatively primitive psychopathology which may be consistent with severe obsessive symptomatology. It suggests, in addition, the need to differentiate between the capacity to establish an analytic situation and the capacity to develop a genuine transference neurosis.

The findings in respect of hysteria were strikingly different. At the time of our follow-up studies, reports tended

> to indicate that hysterical patients, particularly in analysis as first supervised cases, are, to put it simply, very good or very bad patients. . . . Among the hysterical characters, the development of an overt transference neurosis was the rule rather than the exception. . . . Frequently, however, difficulties arise in establishment of the therapeutic alliance. . . . Hysterical patients are, as a rule, readily capable of regressive primary process thinking characteristic of the analytic process. . . . Once a good analytic situation is achieved, hysterics remain potentially the best subjects for classical analytic procedure (Knapp *et al.*, 1960, p. 472).

These findings suggest that it is desirable in considering the criteria for analysability to make a distinction between the analytic situation and the analytic process. It is also helpful to divide clinical psychoanalysis into its three separate phases: first, the initiation and consolidation of the analytic situation; second, the emergence and analysis of the transference neurosis; third, the completion of a successful termination. The analytic situation may be briefly defined as the setting and the continuous mutual identification with a common goal during which intrapsychic changes of a specific nature are mobilized and resolved in the patient. These intrapsychic changes include in essence the emergence and interpretation of the transference neurosis. This comprises the middle stage of analysis. Successful analysis includes, in conclusion, all that is involved in the process of separation and termination.

In considering the criteria for analysability, the capacity of the patient in respect of each of these three phases may be differentiated. Freud's three classical case histories (1905*b*, 1909*a*, 1918) may be cited to illustrate this statement. Let us consider our probable disposal of a contemporary Dora, Rat Man and Wolf Man, referred to an institute for supervised analysis. Apart from her age, which might lead to reservations relevant to the analysis of adolescents, it is highly probable that Dora would promptly be accepted as a classical hysteric, suitable for analysis as a first or second control. It is doubtful that the Rat Man would be so readily accepted. As already indicated, few patients with obsessional symptoms of this severity had been accepted in our Boston sample. He might, however, with certain reservations be considered as a third or fourth control with a specially gifted candidate. It is more probable, however, that he would be referred to an experienced analyst for preliminary therapy or trial analysis. The Wolf Man, finally, would in all probability be considered unsuitable for psychoanalysis without a preliminary period of psychotherapy. These three patients thus cover a wide range from classical symptom hysteria through a relatively severe obsessional neurosis to a patient whose severe symptomatology and character disorder may cover a hidden psychotic core.

Of these three famous patients, however, it is a matter of very general knowledge that the hysterical Dora had the least satisfactory response to the formal requirements of psychoanalysis. Not only did she prematurely terminate her treatment, she also consciously withheld her explicit plans until the very last hour. The Rat Man, in spite of extreme ambivalence, appears to have maintained throughout a high degree of motivation and a considerable capacity for therapeutic alliance. The Wolf Man, despite the tendency to derive passive transference gratification which impeded his progress, responded nevertheless in a predominantly positive way, with considerable symptomatic improvement.

Dora, however, developed neither an overt positive transference neurosis which facilitated passive gratification, nor sufficient motivation towards a therapeutic goal to enable her to withstand her impulses towards repetitive hostile acting out. Therefore, in spite of her theoretical suitability, she proved in practice the least analysable of these three patients. Her case history may be cited as a possible example of the potential good hysteric discussed in Chapter 14. In this group of patients, early establishment of therapeutic alliance often presents technical problems. It is, however, a crucial prerequisite for successful transference analysis.

Dora's later fate, however, also suggests that her pathology might have precluded successful psychoanalytic intervention. It is uncertain how far her fate can, as Freud suggested, be attributed solely to his own failure to recognize and interrupt her emerging transference neurosis. Her early history revealed little if any evidence of a positive relationship or ego identification with her mother. Her subsequent history confirmed a degree of identification with the aggressor which may have impaired the emergence of a genuine triangular conflict. Her continued lifelong tendency to develop and to maintain somatic symptoms suggests a lack of capacity to tolerate anxiety. This may well have played a large part in determining her premature flight from analysis. The marked orality of her presenting symptoms is also in keeping with recent contributions which emphasize the pregenital sources of many hysterical symptoms. Dora may, in summary, have belonged to the group of patients described in Chapter 14 as so-called good hysterics. The response of such patients to traditional analysis must always be regarded with some reserve.

Of these three cases, the Rat Man alone appears to have met this tripartite approach to the criteria of analysability. His capacity for a therapeutic alliance was clear from the outset. Despite his obsessional characteristics, he was able to develop a regressive, highly analysable transference neurosis. This transference is discussed in some detail in Chapter 13. Although his major neurotic defences were clearly obsessional, his symptom formation represented regression from a previously established genital position. In this sense his neurosis, like that of most patients who appear best to meet the criteria for analysability, had both obsessional and hysteric features. Although, finally,

Freud did not present material relevant to the conclusion of the Rat Man's analysis, the fact remains that he was able to terminate. In recent years I have had the opportunity of selecting a few obsessional patients, whose symptoms approached the Rat Man's severity, for analysis under my own supervision. A crucial task in selecting such patients concerns diagnostic evaluation of obsessional symptomatology which, like that of the Rat Man, represents regression from a previously established triangular oedipal situation. This group of patients must be differentiated from the more disturbed patients whose obsessional defences mask a deeper, possibly psychotic disturbance.

My own conscientious objector serves as one illustration of such severe psychopathology. Freud's Wolf Man represents the classic example in analytic literature. His analysis, however, was not a stormy one. Unlike my patient, he was able to utilize the analytic situation as one which gave him considerable gratification. In addition to this analytic stalemate, his reported subsequent history suggests that, like the conscientious objector, he could not be regarded as fully analysable. A question must, however, be raised as to whether patients of this type should always be denied a trial analysis. In spite of later relapses, it may be agreed that the Wolf Man gained immeasurably from his analytic treatment. The fact that our therapeutic goal must be limited in certain patients need not represent an absolute contradiction when and if they are willing to undertake a trial analysis. This, in my opinion, is often the only way to reach a decisive opinion as to the degree and nature of individual psychopathology.

It will be clear from my discussion up to this point that consideration of the criteria for analysability cannot be made without reference to all that is involved in a traditional psychoanalysis. The following chapter, which was originally presented at a panel held at the International Congress in Geneva in July 1955, clearly indicates the degree to which understanding of the nature of the analytic process influences not only technique but also the criteria for recommending analysis. In this chapter explicit reference is made to a term I have emphasized in respect of the analytic situation. This is the term 'therapeutic alliance'. At the time the chapter was originally written such an alliance was mainly attributed to the mature part of the patient's ego.

In subsequent years I have been increasingly impressed by the degree to which the capacity to form a satisfactory therapeutic relationship derives from a relatively early period of life. There has been considerable controversy and difference of opinion regarding this suggestion. The paper 'Therapeutic Alliance in the Psychoanalysis of Hysteria' (Chapter 11) was presented at a meeting of the A.P.A. in 1958. Owing to the confidentiality of the clinical material it was not published at that time. Although, as will be noted in later chapters of this section, I have somewhat expanded my original conception, the basic thesis of this paper remains integral to my present position.

Although the model presented in Chapter 15 is not without certain problems, I nevertheless believe that this chapter presents my current position in a more comprehensive manner than any other included in this volume. This model originated from a doodle stimulated by Maxwell Gitelson's paper 'The Curative Factors in Psychoanalysis' (1962). His thesis closely resembled the arguments I put forward in Chapter 11. In both, an attempt has been made to differentiate the significance of the analytic situation as one which requires affective responses on the part of the analyst from the analyst's position *vis-à-vis* the distortions and regressive wishes which characterize the emergence of the transference neurosis. In trying to formulate my own understanding I reached the conclusion that a developmental approach to psychic life might permit graphic illustration of the difference between basic ego attributes originally acquired in one-to-one relationships, and those intrapsychic defences mobilized by signal anxiety during and after the emergence of the triangular oedipal situation.

The former represents the core of the autonomous ego, operates in an essentially open system and uses neutralized, sublimated or ego-syntonic instinctual energy. The latter represents in essence all that was originally implied by Freud's concept of the repressed unconscious. It thus operates within a relatively closed system unless and until ego defences defined as automatic conscious responses to signal anxiety are significantly threatened. The differences between the classical forms of transference neurosis and more serious pathology attributable to early developmental failure might thus be presented in graphic form.

This model also makes it possible to illustrate the difference between regression limited to the area of unconscious defences in neurotic symptom formation and the transference neurosis, and regression leading to impairment of basic self-esteem or threatening self-object differentiation and the capacity to maintain a one-to-one relationship. This model is thus equally relevant to problems discussed in the first section of the volume and to our understanding of clinical psychoanalysis. It represents one approach to psychoanalysis as a comprehensive developmental psychology.

The thesis underlying the concluding chapter includes some considerations which have recently expanded the argument put forward in respect of the model. Although they are not incompatible, they nevertheless indicate some of the limits inherent in all forms of model-making. The model, for example, does not permit graphic illustration of the differences between one-to-one and triangular object relations. This differentiation is thus implicit rather than explicit in the discussion of all that is involved in the establishment of a relatively closed system. This model has not, in addition, been expanded in respect of the passage of time. It does not thus directly illustrate the reopening of conflict or the ego regression which characterizes the years of adolescence. In this context the increased emphasis placed by many analysts on these regressive features should be noted. If, as Peter Blos (1968) suggests, early pregenital one-to-one conflicts are revived and re-experienced during adolescence, it is hardly surprising that such regression may be a frequent concomitant of clinical psychoanalysis. Recognition of the dyadic object relationship prerequisite to the ego identification achieved during a positive therapeutic alliance need not necessarily imply that the analytic situation represents an explicit revival of the infantile mother–child relationship. However, I would still maintain that analysis, like adolescence, draws on the strengths and reveals the weaknesses of the original developmental process.

All these considerations, and others raised throughout this volume, are included in the last chapter. Here I have attempted to bring together those findings which appear to be most relevant to a psychoanalytic concept of psychic health. Without in any way minimizing the importance of external adaptation and achievement, I have tried to counterbalance these considerations with an equal emphasis on internal factors. I have thus included affect tolerance and mastery as an integral feature of the capacity for emotional growth. In conclusion, I have re-emphasized the crucial importance of a genuine triangular conflict as prerequisite, first, for the emergence of areas of conflict-free interest and ambition, and last but by no means least, for the capacity for meaningful, stable heterosexual relations and a secure sense of sexual identity. Both attributes, it may be suggested, will facilitate emotional growth at each succeeding stage of the life cycle.

10

THE CONCEPT OF TRANSFERENCE[1]

(1956)

There are few current problems concerning the concept of transference that Freud did not recognize either implicitly or explicitly in the development of his theoretical and clinical framework. For all essential purposes, moreover, his formulations, in spite of certain shifts in emphasis, remain integral to contemporary psychoanalytic theory and practice. Recent developments concern the impact of an ego-psychological approach; the significance of object relations, both current and infantile, external and internal; the role of aggression in mental life, and the part played by regression and the repetition compulsion in the transference. Nevertheless analysis of the infantile oedipal situation in the setting of a genuine transference neurosis is still considered the primary goal of traditional psychoanalytic procedure.

Originally, transference was ascribed to displacement on to the analyst of repressed wishes and fantasies derived from early childhood. The transference neurosis was viewed as a compromise formation similar to dreams and other neurotic symptoms. Resistance, defined as the clinical manifestation of repression, could be diminished or abolished by interpretation mainly directed towards the content of the repressed. Transference resistance, both positive and negative, was ascribed to the threatened emergence of repressed unconscious material in the analytic situation. Soon, with the development of a structural approach, the superego, described as the heir to the genital oedipal situation, was also recognized as playing a leading part in the transference situation. The analyst was subsequently viewed not only as the object by displacement of infantile incestuous fantasies, but also as the substitute by projection for

[1] Read at the 19th Congress of the International Psycho-Analytical Association, Geneva, in July 1955. First published in the *Int. J. Psycho-Anal.* (1956), **37**.

the prohibiting parental figures which had been internalized as the definitive superego. The effect of transference interpretation in mitigating undue severity of the superego has been emphasized in many discussions of transference.

Increased recognition of the role of early object relations in the development of both ego and superego has increasingly influenced current concepts of transference. In this connection, the significance of the analytic situation as a repetition of the early mother–child relationship has been stressed from different points of view. An equally important development concerns Freud's revised concept of anxiety which not only led to theoretical developments in the field of ego psychology, but also brought about related clinical changes in the work of many analysts. As a result, attention was no longer primarily focused on the content of the unconscious. In addition, increasing importance was attributed to the defensive processes by means of which anxiety (which would be engendered if repression and other related mechanisms were broken down) was avoided in the analytic situation. Different approaches to the role of the analyst and the nature of transference became increasingly evident. These differences first emerged clearly in discussion of the technique of child analysis, in which Melanie Klein (cf. 1927) and Anna Freud (cf. 1927), the pioneers in this field, played leading roles.

From a theoretical point of view, discussion foreshadowing contemporary problems was presented in well-known papers by Richard Sterba (1934) and James Strachey (1934). Certain points were further elaborated at the Marienbad Symposium at which Edward Bibring (1937) made an important contribution. The importance of identification with, or introjection of, the analyst in the transference situation was clearly indicated. Therapeutic results were attributed to the effect of this process in mitigating the need for pathological defences. Strachey, considerably influenced by the work of Melanie Klein, regarded transference as essentially a projection on to the analyst of the patient's own superego. The therapeutic process was attributed to subsequent introjection of a modified superego as a result of 'mutative' transference interpretation. On the other hand, Sterba and Bibring—intimately involved with development of the ego-psychological approach—emphasized the central role of the ego, postulating a therapeutic split and identification with the analyst as an essential feature of transference.

To some extent, this difference of opinion may be regarded as semantic. If the superego is explicitly defined as the heir of the genital oedipal conflict, then earlier intra-systemic conflicts within the ego, although they may be related retrospectively to the definitive superego, must, nevertheless, be defined as contained within the ego. Later divisions within the ego of the type indicated by Sterba, and much expanded by Bibring in his description of an alliance between the analyst and the healthy part of the patient's ego, are not to be attributed to the definitive superego. In contrast, those who attribute the development of psychic structure primarily to the introjection of part and whole objects have reached the conclusion that the resultant state of internal conflict resembles in all dynamic respects the situation seen in later conflicts between ego and superego. They believe that these structures develop simultaneously, and suggest, therefore, that no sharp distinction should be made between pre-oedipal, oedipal and post-oedipal superego.

The differences, however, are not entirely verbal. Those who attribute superego formation to the early months of life attach a significance to early object relations which differs from the conception of those who regard control and neutralization of instinctual energy as primary functions of the ego. This theoretical difference necessarily implies some disagreement as to the dynamic situation, both in childhood and in adult life. This divergence is inevitably reflected in the concept of transference and in hypotheses as to the nature of the therapeutic process. From one point of view, the role of the ego is central and crucial at every phase of analysis. A differentiation is made between transference as therapeutic alliance and the transference neurosis, which, on the whole, is considered a manifestation of resistance. Effective analysis depends on a sound therapeutic alliance, a prerequisite for which is the integration, before analysis, of certain mature ego functions. These may be absent in certain severely disturbed patients and in young children for whom traditional psychoanalytic procedure may be precluded. Whenever indicated, interpretation must deal with transference manifestations, which clearly implies that the transference must be analysed. The process of analysis, however, is not exclusively to be ascribed to transference interpretation. Other interpretations of unconscious material, whether related to defence or to early fantasy, will be equally effective, provided they are accurately timed and provided a satisfactory therapeutic alliance has been made.

Those, in contrast, who stress the importance of early object relations emphasize the crucial role of transference as an object relationship, distorted though this may be by a variety of defences against primitive unresolved conflicts. The central role of the ego, both in the early stages of development and in the analytic process, is accepted. The nature of the ego is, however, considered at all times to be determined by its external and internal objects. Therapeutic progress indicated by changes in ego function results, therefore, primarily from a change in object relations through interpretation of the transference situation. Little if any differentiation is made between transference as therapeutic alliance and the transference neurosis as a manifestation of resistance. Therapeutic progress, in this view, depends almost exclusively on transference interpretation. Other interpretations, although indicated at times, are not in general considered an essential feature of the analytic process. From this point of view, the pre-analytic maturity of the patient's ego is not stressed as a prerequisite for analysis; children and relatively disturbed patients are considered potentially suitable for traditional psychoanalytic procedure.

These differences in theoretical orientation are not only reflected in the approach to children and disturbed patients. They may also be recognized in significant variations of technique in respect of all clinical groups. These variations inevitably affect the opening phases, the understanding of the inevitable regressive features of the transference neurosis, and the handling of the terminal phases of analysis. I shall try to underline the main problems here by emphasizing contrast rather than similarity. I shall also try to avoid too detailed discussion of controversial theory regarding the nature of early ego development by a somewhat arbitrary differentiation between those who relate ego analysis to the analysis of defences and those who stress the primary significance of object relations, both in the transference and in the development and definitive structure of the ego. While this involves some over-simplification, I hope that it may, at the same time, clarify certain important issues.

To take up first the analysis of patients generally agreed to be suitable for classical analytic procedure, the transference neuroses. Those who emphasize the role of the ego and the analysis of defences not only maintain Freud's conviction that analysis should proceed from surface to depth, but also consider that early material in the analytic situation derives, in general, from defensive processes rather than from displacement on to the analyst of early instinctual fantasies. In the well-defended patient deep transference interpretation in the early phases of analysis may be meaningless to the patient since its unconscious significance is so inaccessible. If, on the other hand, the defences are precarious, such interpretation may lead to premature and possibly intolerable anxiety. Early interpretation of the unconscious automatic defensive processes by means of which instinctual fantasy has been kept unconscious is regarded as equally ineffective and undesirable.

There are, of course, differences of opinion within this group as to how far analysis of defence can be separated from analysis of content. Robert Waelder (1954), for example, has stressed the impossibility of such separation. Otto Fenichel (1941), however, considered that at least theoretical separation should be made, indicating that, as far as possible, analysis of defence should precede analysis of unconscious fantasy. It is nevertheless generally agreed that as a rule the transference neurosis develops after ego defences have been sufficiently undermined to permit mobilization of previously hidden instinctual conflict. During the early stages of analysis, and at frequent points after the development of the transference neurosis, defence against the transference will become a main feature of the analytic situation.

This approach, as already indicated, is based on certain definite premises regarding the nature and function of the ego in controlling and neutralizing instinctual energy and unconscious fantasy. While the importance of early object relations is not neglected, the conviction that early transference interpretation is ineffective and potentially dangerous is related to the hypothesis that the instinctual energy available to the mature ego has been neutralized. At the beginning of analysis, it is thus relatively or absolutely divorced, for all effective purposes, from its unconscious fantasy meaning.

In contrast, there are a number of analysts of different theoretical orientation who do not view the development of the mature ego as a relative separation of ego functions from unconscious sources. They believe that unconscious fantasy continues to operate in all conscious mental activity. These analysts also tend on the whole to emphasize the crucial significance of primitive fantasy in the development of the transference situation. The individual entering analysis will inevitably have unconscious fantasies concerning the analyst, fantasies derived from quite primitive sources. This material, although deep in one sense, is, nevertheless, strongly current and accessible to interpretation. Melanie Klein (1948, 1952), in addition, relates the development and definitive structure of both ego and superego to unconscious fantasy determined by the earliest phases of object relationship. She emphasizes the role of early introjective and projective processes in relation to primitive anxiety ascribed to the death instinct and related aggressive fantasies. In her view, unresolved difficulties and conflicts of the earliest period continue to colour object relations throughout life. Failure to achieve an essentially satisfactory object relationship in this early period is a determinant of failure to retain a good internal object. As a result, relative object loss will not be mastered. Such patterns will not only affect all object relations and definitive ego functions; more specifically, they will determine the nature of anxiety-provoking fantasies on entering the analytic situation. According to this point of view, therefore, early transference interpretation, even though it may relate to fantasies derived from an early period of life, should result not in an increase, but a decrease of anxiety.

In considering problems of transference in relation to analysis of the transference neurosis, two main points must be kept in mind. First, as already suggested, those who emphasize the analysis of defence tend to make a definite differentiation between transference as therapeutic alliance and the transference neurosis as a compromise formation which serves the purposes of resistance. In contrast, those who emphasize the importance of early object relations view the transference primarily as a revival or repetition, sometimes attributed to symbolic processes of early struggles involving object relations. Here, no sharp distinction is made between the early manifestations of transference and the transference neurosis. In view of the weight given to the role of unconscious fantasy and internal objects in every phase of mental life, healthy and pathological mental processes, though differing in their results, do not differ in their direct dependence on primitive unconscious sources.

In the second place, the role of regression in the transference situation is subject to wide differences of opinion. It was, of course, one of Freud's earliest discoveries that regression to earlier points of fixation is a cardinal feature, not only in the development of neurosis and psychosis, but also in the revival of earlier conflicts in the transference situation. With the development of psychoanalysis and its application to an ever-increasing range of disturbed personalities, the role of aggression in the analytic situation has received increased attention. The significance of the analytic situation as a means of fostering regression has been, for example, emphasized by Ida Macalpine (1950), who suggests that such regression is integral to the analytic process.

Differing opinions as to the significance, value and technical handling of regressive manifestations form the basis of important modifications of analytic technique which will be considered presently. With regard to the transference neuroses, the view expressed by Phyllis Greenacre (1954), that regression as an indispensable feature of the transference situation is to be resolved by traditional technique, would be generally accepted. It is also a matter of general agreement that a prerequisite for successful analysis is revival and repetition in the analytic situation of the struggles of primitive stages of development.

Those who emphasize defence analysis, however, tend to view regression as a manifestation of resistance, i.e. as a primitive mechanism of defence employed by the ego in the setting of the transference neurosis. Analysis of these regressive manifestations with their potential dangers depends on the continued functioning of an ego sufficiently strong to maintain therapeutic alliance at an adult level. Those, in contrast, who stress the significance of transference as a revival of the early mother–child relationship do not emphasize regression as an indication of resistance or defence. The revival of these primitive experiences in the transference situation is, in fact, regarded as an essential prerequisite for satisfactory psychological maturation and true genitality. The Kleinian school, as already indicated, stress the continued activity of primitive conflicts in determining essential features of the transference at every stage of analysis. The increasingly overt revival of these conflicts in the analytic situation, therefore, signifies a deepening of the analysis and, in general, is regarded as an indication of diminution rather than increase of resistance. The dangers involved, according to this point of view, are avoided by mitigation of primitive anxiety by suitable transference interpretation. This is far more important than efforts to establish, in the early phases of analysis, a sound therapeutic alliance based on the maturity of the patient's essential ego characteristics.

In considering, however briefly, the terminal phases of analysis, many unresolved problems concerning the goal of therapy and the definition of a completed psychoanalysis must be kept in mind. Distinction must also be made between the technical problems of the terminal phase and evaluation of transference resolution after the analysis has been terminated. There is widespread agreement as to the frequent revival, in the terminal phases, of primitive transference manifestations apparently resolved during the early phase of analysis.

Michael Balint (1952), and those who accept Sándor Ferenczi's concept of primary passive love, suggest that some gratification of primitive passive needs may be essential for successful termination. To Melanie Klein (1950) the terminal phases of analysis also represent such a repetition of important features of the early mother–child relationship; specifically, a revival of the early weaning situation. Completion depends on a mastery of early depressive struggles culminating in successful introjection of the analyst as a good object. Although, in this connection, emphasis differs considerably, it should be noted that those who stress the importance of identification with the analyst as a basis for therapeutic alliance also accept the inevitability of some concomitant permanent modifications. Those who distinguish beween transference and the transference neurosis stress the importance of analysis and resolution of the transference neurosis as a main prerequisite for successful termination. The identification based on therapeutic alliance must be interpreted and understood, particularly with reference to the reality aspects of the analyst's personality. In spite, therefore, of significant important differences, there is, as already indicated in connection with the earlier papers of Sterba and Strachey, considerable agreement as to the goal of psychoanalysis.

The differences already considered indicate some basic current problems of transference. So far, however, discussion has been limited to variations within the framework of a traditional technique. We must now consider problems related to overt modifications. While these variations have been introduced in respect of certain clinical conditions, often as a preliminary to classical psychoanalysis, these must be distinguished from modifications which represent changes in basic approach, and which lead to significant alterations both in the method and in the aim of therapy. It is generally agreed that some variations of technique are indicated in the treatment of certain character neuroses, borderline patients, and the psychoses. The nature and meaning of such changes is, however, viewed differently according to the relative emphasis placed on the ego and its defences, on underlying unconscious conflicts, and on the significance and handling of regression in the therapeutic situation.

In 'Analysis Terminable and Interminable' (1937), Freud suggested that certain ego attributes may be inborn or constitutional and, therefore, probably inaccessible to psychoanalytic procedure. Heinz Hartmann has suggested (Hartmann, 1950, 1952; Hartmann *et al.*, 1946) that in addition to these primary attributes, other ego characteristics originally developed for defensive purposes and the related neutralized instinctual energy at the disposal of the ego, may be relatively or absolutely divorced from unconscious fantasy. Not only does this explain the relative inefficacy of early transference interpretation, it also hints at possible limitations in the potentialities of analysis, limitations which can be ascribed to relatively irreversible secondary autonomy of the ego. In certain cases, moreover, it is suggested that analysis of precarious or seriously pathological defences—particularly those concerned with the control of aggressive impulses—may be not only ineffective, but dangerous. The relative failure of ego development in such cases not only precludes the development of a genuine therapeutic alliance, but also raises the risk of a seriously regressive, often predominantly hostile, transference situation. In certain cases, therefore, a preliminary period of psychotherapy is recommended in order to explore the capacities of the patient to tolerate traditional psychoanalysis. In others, as Robert Knight (1953) in his paper 'Borderline States' and as many analysts working with psychotic patients have suggested, psychoanalytic procedure is not considered applicable. Instead, a therapeutic approach is advocated which is based on analytic understanding and which, in essence, utilizes a positive transference as a means of reinforcing, rather than analysing, the precarious defences of the individual.

In contrast, Herbert Rosenfeld (1952) has treated even severely disturbed psychotic patients with minimal modifications of psychoanalytic technique. The only changes introduced are those necessitated by the severity of the patient's condition. Here, the dangers of regression in therapy are not emphasized, since primitive fantasy is considered to be active under all circumstances. The most primitive period is viewed in terms of early object relations with special stress on persecutory anxiety related to the death instinct. Interpretation of this primitive fantasy in the transference situation, as already indicated, is considered to diminish psychotic anxiety, and thus offer the best opportunity of strengthening the severely threatened psychotic ego.

Other analysts—for example, D. W. Winnicott (1955)—attribute psychosis mainly to severe traumatic experiences, particularly experiences of deprivation in early infancy. According to this point of view, profound regression offers an opportunity to fulfil, in the transference situation, primitive needs which had not been met at the appropriate level of development. Similar suggestions have been proposed by Sidney Margolin (1953) and others in regard to the concept of anaclitic treatment of serious psychosomatic disease. This approach is also based on the premise that the regression inevitably shown by certain patients should be utilized in therapy as a means of gratifying, in an extremely permissive transference situation, demands which had not been met in infancy. It must, in this connection, be noted that the gratifications recommended in the treatment of severely disturbed patients are determined by the conviction that these patients are incapable of developing transference as it is understood in connection with neuroses, and must therefore be handled by a modified technique.

The opinions so far considered, however much they may differ in certain respects, are none the less all based on the premise that the essential difference between analysis and other methods of therapy is whether or not interpretation of transference is an integral feature of technical procedure. Results based on the effects of suggestion are to be avoided, as far as possible, whenever traditional technique is employed. This goal has, however, proved more difficult to achieve than Freud expected when he first discerned the significance of symptomatic recovery based on positive transference. The importance of suggestion, even in the most strict analytic methods, has been repeatedly stressed by Edward Glover (1954, 1955) and others. Increasing emphasis on the part played by the analyst's personality in determining the course of the individual transference implies recognition of unavoidable suggestive tendencies inherent in the therapeutic process. Many analysts today believe that the classical ideal of analytic objectivity and anonymity cannot be maintained. Instead, thorough analysis of reality aspects of the therapist's personality and point of view is advocated as an essential feature of transference analysis, and as an indispensable prerequisite for the dynamic changes already discussed in relation to the termination of analysis. It thus remains the ultimate goal of psychoanalysts, whatever their theoretical orientation, to avoid results based on the unrecognized or unanalysed action of suggestion. They maintain, as their primary goal, the resolution of such results through consistent and careful interpretation.

There are, however, a number of therapists, both within and outside the field of psychoanalysis, who hold that the transference situation should not be regarded solely or primarily as a setting for interpretation even in the treatment or analysis of neurotic patients. Instead, they advocate utilization of the transference relationship for the manipulation of corrective emotional experience. The theoretical orientation of those utilizing the concept of transference may be closer to, or more distant from, a Freudian point of view according to the degree to which current relationships are seen as determined by past events. At one extreme, current aspects and cultural factors are considered of predominant importance; at the other, mental development is viewed in essentially Freudian terms. Modifications of technique are seen as necessary because of limitations inherent in the analytic method. They are not attributed to essentially changed conceptions of the early phases of mental development.

Of this group, Franz Alexander (1950) is perhaps the best example. In his Salzburg paper (1925), he had indicated the tendency for patients—even after apparently successful transference analysis of the oedipal situation—to regress to narcissistic dependent, pregenital levels. This state of affairs often proves to be stubborn and refractory to transference interpretation. In his more recent work, the role of regression in the transference situation has been increasingly stressed. The emergence and persistence of dependent, pregenital demands in a very wide range of clinical conditions, it is argued, indicate that the encouragement of a regressive transference situation is undesirable and therapeutically ineffective. The analyst therefore should, when regression threatens, adopt a definite role explicitly differing from the behaviour of the parents in early childhood. This may bring about therapeutic results through a corrective emotional experience in the transference situation. Such procedures, it is suggested, may obviate the tendency to regression, thus curtailing the length of treatment and improving therapeutic results. According to this point of view, limitation of regressive manifestations by such active steps which modify traditional analytic procedure in a variety of ways is frequently indicated.

It will be clear that to those who are convinced that interpretation of all transference manifestations remains an essential feature of psychoanalysis, the type of modification here described, even though based on a Freudian reconstruction of the early phases of mental development, represents a major change. This modification is motivated by the belief that psychoanalysis as a therapeutic method has limitations which are linked to the tendency to regression, and which cannot be resolved by traditional technique. Moreover, the fundamental premise on which the conception of corrective emotional experience is based minimizes the significance of insight and recall. It is, essentially, suggested that corrective emotional experience alone may bring about qualitative dynamic alterations in mental structure, alterations which can then lead to a satisfactory therapeutic goal. This implies a definite modification of the analytic hypothesis that current problems are determined by the defences against instinctual impulses and/or internalized objects which had been set up during the decisive periods of early development. In the traditional view, a genuine analytic result depends on the revival, repetition and mastery of earlier conflicts in the current experience of the transference situation, with insight regarded as an indispensable feature of the analytic goal.

Since certain important modifications are related to the concept of regression in the transference situation, I should like briefly to consider this concept in relation to the repetition compulsion. That transference, essentially a revival of earlier emotional experience, must be regarded as a manifestation of the repetition compulsion, is generally accepted. It is, however, necessary to distinguish between repetition compulsion as an attempt to master traumatic experience and repetition compulsion as an attempt to return to a real or fantasied earlier state of rest or gratification. Daniel Lagache (1951) has related the repetition compulsion to an inherent need to return to any problem previously left unsolved. From this point of view, the regressive aspects of the transference situation are to be regarded as a necessary preliminary to the mastery of unresolved conflict. From a second point of view, however, the regressive aspects of transference are mainly attributed to a wish to return to an earlier state of rest or narcissistic gratification, to the maintenance of the *status quo* in preference to any progressive action, and finally, to Freud's original conception of the death instinct. There is a good deal to suggest that both aspects of the repetition compulsion may be seen in the regressive aspects of every analysis. To those who feel that regressive self-destructive forces tend to be stronger than progressive libidinal impulses, the potentialities of the analytic approach will inevitably appear to be limited. Those, in contrast, who regard the reappearance in the transference situation of earlier conflicts as an indication of tendencies to master and progress will continue to feel that the classical analytic method remains the optimal approach to psychological illness wherever it is applicable.

To conclude: I have tried in this chapter to outline some current problems of transference, both in relation to the history of psychoanalytic thought and in relation to the theoretical premises on which they are based. With regard to contemporary views which advocate serious modification of analytic technique, I cannot improve on the remarks made by Ernest Jones in his introduction to the Salzburg Symposium: 'depreciation of the Freudian (infantile) factors at the expense of the pre-Freudian ones (pre-infantile and post-infantile) is a highly characteristic manifestation of the general human resistance against the acceptance of the importance of the former, being usually a flight from the Oedipus complex which is the centre of infantile factors. We also know that the practice of psychoanalysis does not always ensure immunity from this reaction' (1925, p. 3). With regard to the important problems which arise from genuine scientific differences within the framework of traditional technique, I have tried to focus the issues for discussion by emphasizing as objectively as possible divergence rather than agreement. I should like, however, to end on a more personal note. I have had unusual opportunities to observe at close quarters impressive achievements by analysts of widely divergent theoretical orientation in different parts of the world. All of them agree as to the primary importance of transference analysis. None have accepted any significant modifications of traditional technique as a means of either shortening analysis or accepting a modified analytic goal. Finally, all agree as to the basic importance of understanding the significance and possible dangers of countertransference manifestations. Unfortunately, however, this vitally important unconscious reaction is not limited to the individual analytic situation. It may also be aroused by scientific theories both within and outside our special field of knowledge. Just as resolution of the individual transference situation depends on the analyst's understanding of his own countertransference, so, too, similar insight and objectivity on a wider scale may lead to resolution of the problems outlined.

11

THERAPEUTIC ALLIANCE IN THE ANALYSIS OF HYSTERIA[1]

(1958)

At the core of clinical psychoanalysis is the revival and subsequent resolution of the main infantile conflict situations in the setting of the transference neurosis. It is a fundamental prerequisite for the analytic undertaking that the analyst should maintain an attitude of objectivity and neutrality towards the distortions and projections which inevitably arise. It is also generally recognized that, over and above the transference neurosis, successful analysis demands at its nucleus a consistent, stable relationship which will enable the patient to maintain an essentially positive attitude towards the analytic task when the conflicts revived in the transference neurosis bring disturbing wishes and fantasies close to the surface of consciousness.

In his early technical papers Freud clearly described this nucleus of the therapeutic relationship as a well-developed rapport. In 'Analysis Terminable and Interminable' he defined it in structural terms: 'As is well known, the analytic situation consists in our allying ourselves with the ego of the person under treatment, in order to subdue portions of his id which are uncontrolled—that is to say to include them in the synthesis of his ego' (1937, p. 235). Therapeutic alliance may be defined as a working relationship between patient and analyst. During the course of analytic work, a split in the ego of the patient takes place along the lines described by Richard Sterba (1934) and Edward Bibring (1937). This split allows the mature or observing part of the patient's ego to identify with the analyst in the task of modifying pathological defences previously set up against internal danger situations. In addition, since two participants are inevitably involved, it is clear that analytic progress must in some respects depend on an object relationship.

[1] Adapted from a paper presented at a meeting of the American Psychoanalytic Association in 1958.

The nature of this object relationship has, in general, been approached from two points of view. In terms of mature ego functions and reality testing, the ability of the patient to maintain a real relationship with the analyst as a separate individual—with both positive and negative attributes—appears to be related to his capacity for therapeutic alliance. In this connection it is recognized that the analyst's real personality and individual characteristics inevitably influence the analytic situation. Anna Freud, in her discussion at the Arden House meetings (1954), affirmed the importance of the analyst as a real person in the analytic process. Recognition and interpretation of this aspect of the analytic situation must, of course, be clearly differentiated from over-active or inappropriate participation on the part of the analyst. Grete Bibring, in a paper entitled 'A Contribution to the Subject of Transference Resistance' (1936), indicated how, in certain situations, real characteristics of the analyst may militate against the achievement of a basic relationship between patient and analyst which is sufficiently positive to permit satisfactory working through and resolution of the transference neurosis.

It has also been widely suggested that at the heart of transference is a relationship recapitulating crucial aspects of the early mother–child relationship. Phyllis Greenacre, for example, has posited the existence of a 'matrix' of transference (1958). Hans Loewald, in his papers 'Ego and Reality' (1951) and 'On the Therapeutic Action of Psychoanalysis' (1960), argues for a similar point of view. It is important to realize, however, that many of these contributions (for this issue, cf. Ferenczi, Balint, Spitz, Hoffer and Klein) refer to this fundamental nucleus transference in terms of its most primitive implications. Sándor Ferenczi and Michael Balint, in particular, have proposed that the analyst should assume a gratifying maternal role. In the important analogies he has drawn between sleep, the dream and the analytic situation, Bertram Lewin (1954) refers to the tendency to regress to an extremely primitive level at which the oral triad is dominant, a stage which precedes the development of true object relations and the beginning of a sense of separate identity. Ives Hendrick (1942, 1951) has suggested in this connection that a differentiation should be made between the earliest object relationships, which are essentially dyadic, and the oedipal situation, which is triangular or triadic. Since successful analysis demands not only resolution of the crucial triangular situation, but, in addition, revival and repetition of earlier pregenital conflicts, it follows that the transference neurosis will inevitably evoke both triadic and dyadic manifestations.

In connection with the earlier period, however, an essential distinction must be made between the earliest mother–child relationship as a symbiosis in which ego boundaries have not been delineated, in which primary identification is dominant, and in which archaic fantasies of omnipotence prevail, and the period after the child has reached the stage at which early reality testing and the first sustained object relationships should be achieved. It is at this level, while still in the setting of predominantly one-to-one relationships, that the child must master his responses of rage and anxiety in the face of frustration; that he first differentiates between external and internal danger situations; that he gains awareness of his own identity as separate from that of his object and first enjoys the acquisition of independent skills and understanding—a process which involves mechanisms of secondary identification—and, finally, that he learns to accept a degree of dependence without demanding total gratification. The achievement of a positive sustained relationship with an underlying attitude of trust, in the sense described by Erik Erikson (1950), is critically important for the development of a mature ego capable of good object relationships. The definitive achievement of a mature identity, however, depends on a continuing struggle marked by a series of crises which, albeit with new modifications, revive and repeat the initial conflicts. From the onset of the oedipal period, although crucial problems may be predominantly experienced in a complex triadic form, there nevertheless remains a dyadic element in every situation of frustration and anxiety, which significantly influences its outcome. The less successful the outcome of the initial struggle, the greater, in later conflict situations, will be the regressive tendency towards levels preceding delineation of ego boundaries.

In this respect, the analytic situation may be regarded as a special controlled conflict situation. Resolution of psychic distress in this therapeutically induced conflict is contingent on sufficient success, at a pre-oedipal level, for the patient to establish and maintain a secure basic relationship which recognizes the integrity of separate individuals. This forms the basis of the therapeutic alliance which demands as prerequisite the capacity to tolerate anxiety and frustration, to accept certain reality limitations, and to differentiate between the mature and infantile aspects of mental life. This relationship acts, on the one hand, as a barrier to significant ego regression, and, on the other, as a fundamental feature of the analytic situation against which the fantasies, memories and emotions evoked by the transference neurosis can be measured and contrasted. The achievement and maintenance of this relationship present a wide range of clinical problems, for they depend not only on the psychopathology of the patient but also on the stage of analysis under consideration. In many character neuroses, borderline conditions and in severe neurotic disorders it may be difficult, if not impossible, to make either a theoretical or a clinical distinction between therapeutic alliance as a real object relationship and the appearance of the transference neurosis. During the course of every successful analysis, moreover, therapeutic alliance must eventually evolve into transference analysis if the patient is to achieve an optimal level of maturity and capacity for object relations.

On the one hand, then, therapeutic alliance depends on the successful mobilization of ego characteristics on which depends the capacity for object relationships and reality testing. There are, of course, technical considerations as to the means by which the analyst may best elicit the patient's underlying capacities to create and maintain a secure underlying, reality-orientated object relationship, a relationship which must withstand the inevitable distortions and regressive features of the transference neurosis. On the other hand, in so far as the ego capacities involved are integrally related to pregenital conflicts experienced in an essentially one-to-one relationship, it must also be recognized that when analysis approaches this level, the very relationship which could at one stage of analysis be fostered as the basis of therapeutic alliance must itself enter the domain of transference analysis. It is, in short, inevitable that at some point certain fundamental features of the analytic situation, usually ascribed to therapeutic alliance, become integral to the analysis of the transference neurosis. Since, moreover, it is suggested that the core of therapeutic alliance derives from conflicts experienced at a pregenital level, it follows that it is predominantly in the transference analysis of dyadic object relationships that the distinction between transference neurosis and therapeutic alliance becomes increasingly difficult to maintain.

In clinical work, therefore, the following premises are of importance. First, it is important in the psychoanalysis of patients considered suitable for classical psychoanalytic procedure to make a distinction between therapeutic alliance, defined as a real object relationship which fosters mobilization of autonomous ego attributes in the patients, and the transference neurosis, in which the analyst is utilized as the displaced object of unresolved infantile fantasy. Second, this differentiation will be most evident in the analysis of patients whose initial transference material is expressed in predominantly triadic (that is to say, oedipal) manifestations. Third, the ego capacities which in the early stages of analysis facilitate and foster the development of therapeutic alliance of such patients must themselves enter the sphere of transference analysis, in so far as the analysis is pursued to pregenital conflicts which concern the acceptance of reality and the development of object relations.

The differentiation between the creation and maintenance of therapeutic alliance in the early stages of analysis, and the fact that this relationship must involve transference interpretation if analysis is to be successfully terminated, is particularly relevant to the analysis of neurotic patients who do not present gross disturbances of reality testing prior to analysis. The analysis of hysterical patients is in this respect particularly instructive. On the one hand, the initial transference neurosis of hysterical patients is typically composed of unmistakably oedipal material. Yet, on the other, the underlying oral genesis of hysterical disorders, as is increasingly recognized, makes it necessary to emphasize the establishment, in the early stages of analysis, of a therapeutic alliance which simultaneously utilizes available mature ego resources and limits premature regressive developments. In the terminal stages of analysis, moreover, it has become increasingly clear that resolution of conflicts initially presented at an oedipal level is contingent on analysis of much earlier conflicts—the accomplishment of object relationships which involve acceptance of reality and its limitations.

In order at this point is a review of hysterical patients potentially capable of achieving a therapeutic alliance sufficiently stable to permit full analysis of the transference neurosis. The emphasis here is less on the pathology of the patient and more on the technique of the analysis. Some of the crucial questions which must be considered are: how may the analyst foster the progress of the analysis on the one hand, and, on the other, how may he limit the development of a seriously regressive transference neurosis? What, in short, is the analyst's role in the development of therapeutic alliance? How is this activity to be distinguished from countertransference? How may this alliance be maintained at the height of an intense transference neurosis? How, finally, do interpretation and analysis of the object relationship, implicit to therapeutic alliance, influence resolution in the terminal stages of analysis?

For the first and almost the only time prior to the terminal phases of analysis, patient and analyst meet in the initial interviews and the arrangements for treatment in a predominantly one-to-one relationship: a relationship relatively undisturbed by an overt transference neurosis and the regressive tendencies soon to be fostered by the analytic situation. It is important in this connection that a differentiation should be made, with respect to practical recommendations and to the accepted attitudes of psychoanalysts, between the reality situations which confronted pioneer analysts and that which faces us today. In order that psychoanalysis should develop, it was clearly essential that such fundamental features as regular attendance, prompt payment and, above all, predominant emphasis on the transference neurosis as a relationship in which the analyst did not participate, should be firmly maintained. A new and powerful therapeutic method, which depended on the establishment and resolution of a relationship qualitatively different from any other, was then a-building, despite widespread disapproval and opposition. It was in this setting that Freud said:

> In regard to time, I adhere strictly to the principle of leasing a definite hour [to each patient] . . . it belongs to him and he is liable for it, even if he does not make use of it (1913*a*, p. 126).
>
> I cannot advise my colleagues too urgently to model themselves during psychoanalytic treatment on the surgeon, who puts aside all

his feelings, even his human sympathy, and concentrates his mental forces on the single aim of performing the operation as skilfully as possible (1912, p. 115).

Such statements of general principle were based on Freud's recognition of the specific qualities of the transference neurosis and the means by which its development could be safeguarded. They did not, in practice, exclude the development of a secure working relationship between patient and analyst.

The reality situation today is very different. The principles and practice of psychoanalysis are far more widely accepted, at least at a conscious level. The majority of analytic patients value their place on the couch as a hard-won privilege. From this point of view it is no longer absolutely essential to adhere to rigid rules of procedure. Nevertheless, the wide expansion of psychotherapeutic techniques in recent years has created new problems. Many such techniques permit a more explicit, overt relationship between doctor and patient than is consistent with psychoanalysis of a transference neurosis. It has become necessary to make a clear distinction between the aims and technique of psychotherapy and of psychoanalysis. To a significant degree, a tendency has developed to characterize this differentiation by the relative lack of the analyst's participation and interaction with the analytic patient. Otherwise warm and friendly psychiatrists often adopt in the analytic situation an attitude of silence and uncompromising rigidity. This may be attributed to two main sources. First, it may be the analyst's conviction that any real relationship between patient and himself should be rigorously avoided; second, he may be unable to differentiate, in the early hours of treatment, between material indicative of anxiety and insecurity in the analytic situation (anxiety which, as a rule, accompanies the establishment of therapeutic alliance) and more specific material adumbrating the transference neurosis proper. There is general agreement that the transference neurosis tends to develop gradually and that premature interpretation may have unfortunate results. It is, however, my increasing conviction (particularly with respect to the supervised analysis of hysterical patients) that serious problems in subsequent transference analysis may frequently be attributed to failure to achieve a secure therapeutic alliance by appropriate interpretative intervention in the initial phases of treatment.

The role of therapeutic alliance in the analysis of hysteria may be illustrated in relation to three aspects of treatment. Clinical material will be cited in respect of, first, its opening phases; second, the role of therapeutic alliance during the emergence of the transference neurosis; and third, the influence of interpretation and analysis of the object relationship implicit in therapeutic alliance during the terminal phases of analysis. Three patients are described in this chapter. Each of these patients subsequently resolved the oedipal conflicts which led her to seek therapeutic analysis. None of these patients was seriously disabled except in the area of heterosexual object relations at the time they commenced treatment. In each case the major presenting symptoms justified a presumptive diagnosis of hysteria. As will be noted, however, each of these patients demonstrated unresolved problems in respect of the early mother–child relationship. Each showed regressive tendencies relatively early in analysis. For each of them, therefore, the establishment and maintenance of therapeutic alliance were of crucial importance. The technical steps which proved to be helpful will be indicated and discussed in connection with each of these case illustrations.

To illustrate: one patient reported in her first hour that she had spent the weekend looking for something to do. She had felt lonely. Wherever she went, people seemed to be sad. She had attended a conference at which a number of well-known psychologists had been on the platform. The audience seemed pathetic and one-half crackpots. She wondered if she were one of them. She focused on one woman in particular. She thought the speakers might be laughing at the audience. Maybe, she concluded, it was all her.

This patient's anxiety about entering analysis, and about appearing contemptible or ridiculous, was close to the surface of this material. The first few hours produced considerable additional material of a similar nature, revealing the patient's increasing tendency to view the rather silent analyst as an unreal, omnipotent figure. The patient felt threatened by feelings of utter helplessness against which she defended herself by denial and some displacement. After discussing the situation in his supervisory session, the candidate concerned became aware of his rigidity and concern lest any activity on his part should be regarded as unanalytic in respect of this, his first analytic patient. He adopted subsequently a slightly more active and human attitude, indicating to the patient his recognition of her anxiety. As a result the patient reported the next day that until yesterday she had thought of the analyst as a distant, Olympian, somewhat magical figure. If, for example, he were taking notes these must be written on a special pad, with a special pen which would make no noise. Now she realized that this picture had been fantastic. He was, after all, an ordinary man. If he were taking notes it would be on an ordinary pad with an ordinary pen.

It should be emphasized that this patient, who entered analysis because of inhibitions in her heterosexual relationships (which appeared to be predominantly hysterical), was not seriously disturbed. She functioned extremely well in her professional life and in relatively superficial personal relationships. She had an unusual degree of psychological insight and was highly motivated towards the psychoanalytic task. The rapid emergence of material related to reality testing, with fantasies depicting the analytic relationship as involving an omnipotent analyst and a helpless patient, illustrates the underlying primitive residuum of many hysterical disorders. In the very first hour, moreover, this patient referred to her mother, describing her as a hoarder. Within a few hours she explicitly identified her analyst with the most negative aspects of her father's personality. It has long been recognized that the material produced in the first hours of analysis is frequently extremely revealing, since it foreshadows to a considerable extent the future development of the transference neurosis. For many reasons, early transference interpretation of such material is inappropriate. As this material indicates, however, complete silence and lack of participation may also foster the development of a regressive transference neurosis and impede the growth of the real relationship with which we have contrasted it. If the analyst can actively convey his participation and partnership with the patient as a real person, development of a secure working relationship—the therapeutic alliance—will be encouraged. This participation is essential for the emergence of an analysable transference neurosis in which the triadic oedipal conflict may first be revived at a predominantly genital level. It is only after considerable progress in development of the partnership has been made that analytic resolution of the more primitive core may be attempted.

In the opening hours of analysis, certain hysterical patients tend, on the one hand, rapidly to identify the analyst with pathological characteristics of their original parental figures, and, on the other hand, reveal a vulnerability in reality testing which indicates disturbance at a deep, pregenital level. In the course of supervising candidates' control cases and of conducting clinical conferences, I have had contact with many such cases. One particular group raises theoretical and clinical problems about the role of therapeutic alliance. These patients, like the one described above, were all essentially hysterical, single young women, who entered analysis with a male therapist, mainly because of difficulties in establishing rewarding heterosexual relationships—none, at the time of entering analysis, had such a relationship on a sustained basis. All developed an intense sexualized early transference neurosis, simultaneously initiating a potentially serious relationship with a man who had previously been viewed indifferently. All attempted within six months of beginning treatment to draw the analyst into an overt rivalry situation, indicating in dreams, in associations and in symptomatic behaviour the degree to which the analyst had been utilized as the displaced object of unconscious oedipal fantasies.

The analytic outcome of the common technical problems which developed was, of course, determined to a considerable extent by differences in the character structure of the patients, their motivation and the history of their previous object relations. It is obvious that unresolved problems affecting the analyst's countertransference must increase such problems. Quite apart from these factors, however, it has been my repeated impression that, as the transference neurosis develops, the analytic outcome is to a considerable extent influenced by the relationship achieved in the initial phases of treatment. If, for example, the original arrangements about time and fees have not been settled on a reality basis, taking into account the individual needs and requirements of both participants; if, in addition, the analyst has not in the early stages of analysis dealt adequately with the patient's initial anxieties; if, finally, the analyst is unable as the transference neurosis develops to show the patient a distinction between her oedipal fantasies and the real relationship, the regressive tendencies already described are likely to be seriously intensified. The transference neurosis, although expressed in genital terms, will reveal increasingly primitive features. The patient, unable to tolerate the frustrations and limitations imposed by the analytic situation, will manifest increasing difficulty in maintaining ego boundaries, with an increase in the tendency to serious acting out.

If, by way of contrast, the initial contact and the responses in the early hours have been adequate, the analyst will be better able as the transference neurosis develops to maintain therapeutic alliance and to mobilize the mature portion of the patient's ego. For example, one patient revealed in the first hour an intense need for approval and a tendency to identify the analyst with a highly pathological father with whom there had been considerable mutual involvement. This young woman, in the first six weeks of analysis, displaced much of her transference neurosis to a young man who wanted to marry her. She tended, in this connection, to set up an absolute dichotomy between the analytic situation and the outside relationship. Both Ted and the analyst demanded of her total submission and acceptance. At the same time she was aware that she had manipulated Ted by devices characteristic of her previous heterosexual relationships, and warned the analyst not to get too close to her. At one juncture, Ted made arrangements which would interfere with an analytic hour, a situation which the patient presented to the analyst in an absolute fashion. Either she went to the theatre with Ted, which might mean giving up the analysis, or she sacrificed Ted for the analytic hour. The analyst, quite properly, commented on the absolute form in which the situation was presented. In her subsequent associations it became clear that Ted had, in fact, demanded that she give up analysis. She also reported an intense transference dream. In this dream, she had come for her analytic hour, and the analyst had told her he could not continue to analyse her because he had fallen in love with her. She had then informed Ted that she was not in love with him. The patient found the dream embarrassing; it was also disturbing because it brought so clearly to the fore her need to manipulate men. The analyst interpreted her tendency to set up absolute situations as an indication both of her need to manipulate and of her deeper hope that she might not succeed. A distinction was made between the oedipal content of the dream and her more mature desire that the analyst should resemble neither her omnipotent father nor her devalued mother. He should, rather, become a different parental figure who would help her to achieve and maintain her own identity as a separate person by freeing her from her underlying conviction that external approval was absolutely essential. After a brief period of conflict the patient took a definitive step, deciding not to become engaged. The analysis continued on the basis of a more stable therapeutic alliance.

This case indicates how, in the development of an intense sexualized transference neurosis, a therapeutic alliance based on recognition of ego boundaries and objective reality testing may limit serious regressive tendencies and significant acting out. In addition, it illustrates certain aspects of hysteria which are particularly relevant to the significance of therapeutic alliance as an object relationship. In the case of this girl, as in several others in this group, there was a good deal to indicate that the unconscious incestuous attitude of the father had been a significant factor in the psychogenesis of this patient's symptomatology. In addition to disturbances of genital functions, there were deeper disturbances in the capacity for object relations, reality testing and the maintenance of ego boundaries. In a paper entitled 'Reality Trauma and Reality Sense' read at the London Congress in 1953, I discussed a group of hysterical patients who had shown regressive, reality-distorting responses to gross overt traumatic events in the latency period. In each of these cases, earlier problems in object relations and reality testing proved a significant factor in the patient's response to post-oedipal traumatic experiences. There is reason to believe that this finding has a wider application, particularly relevant to the psychopathology and psychoanalysis of hysteria. Failure at a primitive level to accept the limitations of reality, to progress from primary to secondary mechanisms of identification, and to delineate ego boundaries, leads to increased sensitivity (particularly at the oedipal level) to the unconscious emotional attitudes of parental figures. Subsequent failure to resolve the oedipal situation will predispose such individuals to hysterical disorders. At the same time, mutual involvement of parent and child will tend, as in the case just described, to confirm and reinforce unconscious fantasies of omnipotence which had not been relinquished at an earlier period. Such patients all too readily identify the analyst with the more pathological aspects of their original parental figures. Many of them, however (like both of the patients described), in spite of the relative failure which makes them vulnerable, possess ego strength sufficient to allow the achievement of real object relationships, and the maintenance of an adequate therapeutic alliance in transference analysis.

As analysis proceeds towards the resolution of the transference neurosis, dreams and fantasies often demonstrate the movement of the analysis into its terminal phases. Initially such material is typically progressive rather than regressive. To give one very brief clinical example: The patient was a hysterical young woman, whose femininity had previously been impaired by her deep identification with a disturbed, inadequate mother. During the early stages of analysis she had experienced considerable difficulty in achieving a stable therapeutic alliance with her woman analyst. During this process, however, it had become clear that her early development had been substantially successful. Both her symptoms and her hysterical character traits had followed severe traumatic experiences at the height of her infantile neurosis. Subsequent to these events her mother appears to have suffered a gradual deterioration, characterized by depression and failure in the mother–daughter relationship. Shortly before the dream in question she had met the man who became her husband after termination of the analysis. The dream was as follows: She is with a woman, possibly her mother, but she is not quite sure because she does not look like her. They are in some sort of summer pavilion. Somebody gives her mother a box. The patient looks at the box and sees that it is not one but two identical boxes. This woman gives the patient one of these boxes which then turns out to be a beautiful leather handbag or travelling case with costly and new gold fittings.

This dream indicated a modification of the earlier identification with her devalued mother, through a positive secondary identification with her woman analyst. The initiation of separateness and genuine autonomy was exemplified by the fact that not one, but two objects symbolizing female genitality were available. The patient's analysis was thus entering its terminal stage. This period included, first, a more progressive working through of the transference neurosis. Though the themes dealt with were not new, significant integration of her feminine identification could clearly be noted. At the same time the terminal phases of this analysis were also characterized by depression, separation anxiety, and other regressive features. This, as is well known, is integral to the terminal period of every successful analysis. This patient was nevertheless able to terminate her analysis less than a year after she reported this dream. She has subsequently married, surmounting without regression an ectopic pregnancy, after which she gave birth to a son following an uncomplicated pregnancy. Though she has moved to another city she still writes to her analyst on important occasions. A more detailed clinical example describing such regression and emphasizing the importance of tolerance and mastery of depression during the terminal stages of analysis is presented in Chapter 6.

In this chapter the therapeutic alliance has been considered in its particular relevance to the psychoanalysis of hysteria. The following points may be mentioned in summary. First, over and above the transference neurosis a relationship must exist which enables the patient to differentiate between objective reality and the distortions and projections excited by that neurosis. Second, since this relationship is frequently tempered by current objective external reality, the real personality features of the analyst must be given full consideration. Third, the capacity to form the necessary relationship—therapeutic alliance—on which the crucial differentiation depends, originates at an essentially pregenital level. Fourth, as transference analysis impinges on the basic conflicts in question, transference neurosis and therapeutic alliance tend to merge to a degree which may make them indistinguishable. In essence, I have proposed what might be described as a dual approach to transference, emphasizing the differentiation which must be maintained throughout analysis between dyadic and triadic aspects of the transference situation.

In so far as the therapeutic alliance derives from an early stage in the development of object relations and reality testing, the period during which the child has made decisive steps towards the achievement of a separate identity must be considered of crucial importance. It should be stressed in this connection that parental encouragement of the child's efforts towards independence is as important in the later stages of infantile development as is the provision of security and gratification at the early levels. A relationship of mutual trust and understanding, in which the inevitability of limitations, frustrations and disappointments is understood and accepted by both participants, originates in early childhood, when the child first achieves the nucleus of his separate identity. Certain failures in early development not only predispose the individual to hysterical problems at an oedipal level, but in addition increase the likelihood of a seriously regressive transference neurosis. Although successful termination must involve revival of primitive conflicts regarding object relationships, it is an essential prerequisite that a relatively mature object relationship should first be achieved and maintained in order to avoid fruitless regression to a level at which reality resting may be seriously impaired. Maintenance of this relationship will facilitate the emergence of primitive material which may without undue ego regression be contrasted with reality, for to conclude with a quotation from 'Analysis Terminable and Interminable': 'We must not forget that the analytic relationship is based on a love of truth—that is, on a recognition of reality' (1937, p. 248).

12

THE ANALYTIC SITUATION AND THE ANALYTIC PROCESS[1]

(1966–69)

Psychotherapy, as Freud reminded us over sixty years ago, is the most ancient form of treatment in medicine.

> Certain diseases . . . are far more readily accessible to mental influences than to any other form of medication. It is not a modern dictum but an old saying of physicians that these diseases are not cured by the drug but by the physician, that is, by the personality of the physician, inasmuch as through it he exerts a mental influence (1905*a*, p. 259).

This manifest accessibility may be said to have shaped the destiny of the neurotics in so far as they were to become the patients who would demonstrate the value, the limitations and the dangers of psychotherapy and psychoanalysis. The attitude of expectant faith, as Freud soon discovered, though it sometimes fostered improvement, did not lead to permanent cure. When the dynamic nature of repression was elucidated, the cause of neurosis was attributed to unconscious mental content. As the psychoanalytic method developed, the real personality of the physician became blurred, overshadowed or even lost as the sexualized transference neurosis took the centre of the stage.

It was, of course, a milestone in the development of psychoanalysis when Freud recognized this new compromise formation,

[1] Adapted from two papers: (1) 'The Analytic Situation', presented at the First Pan-American Congress for Psychoanalysis in March 1964 and first published in *Psychoanalysis in the Americas*, edited by Robert E. Litman (New York: International Universities Press, 1966); and (2) 'The Analytic Process', presented at the Second Pan-American Congress for Psychoanalysis in August 1966 and first published in *Psicoanális en las Américas*, edited by L. Grinberg, M. Langer and E. Rodrigué (Buenos Aires: Editorial Paidós, 1969).

designed to serve the forces of resistance. This was not based primarily on emotions appropriate to the current doctor–patient relationship, but derived from wishes, fantasies and memories which had been repressed by intrapsychic forces within the patient's mental apparatus. It was this insight which led to the constructive use of interpretation as the major tool of clinical psychoanalysis. Interpretation, however, could only be effective if the analyst maintained distance and objectivity. Active support, praise, suggestions and advice might lead to emotional involvement (i.e. countertransference). By 1912, therefore, Freud said: 'Emotional coldness in the analyst . . . creates the most advantageous conditions for both parties: for the doctor a desirable protection for his own emotional life and for the patient the largest amount of help we can give him today' (1912, p. 115).

In an almost contemporaneous paper, however, Freud also stated:

> It remains the first aim of the treatment to attach [the patient] to it and to the person of the doctor . . . . If one exhibits a serious interest in him, carefully clears away the resistances that crop up at the beginning and avoids making certain mistakes, he will of himself form such an attachment and link the doctor up with one of the imagos of the people by whom he was accustomed to be treated with affection (1913*a*, p. 139).

This statement suggests that a real doctor–patient relationship was still recognized as an indispensable feature of the analytic situation, a concept which was reinforced in the paper's conclusion: 'The primary motive force is the patient's suffering and the wish to be cured' (1913*a*, p. 143).

Freud defined his recommendation of coldness as optimal 'at that time', suggesting that he himself may have foreseen some potential future changes. His references, moreover, to support and to positive feeling clearly indicate his intuitive awareness that psychoanalysis required more than interpretation of the transference neurosis. His case histories, particularly the analysis of the Rat Man, also reveal his constant response to his patient as a whole person. Though the analytic work concentrated on interpretation of the transference neurosis, this would have been impossible without the clear separation of transference from reality, the mutual alliance towards a therapeutic goal, and the genuine object relationship which remained intact despite the expression by the patient of ambivalence, hostility and intense resistance.

Both the technique and the theory of clinical psychoanalysis have been based, from the outset, on a hypothetical model of the psychic apparatus. This model originally derived from the observations made in the analysis of neurotic patients and from dream interpretation which led Freud to postulate a dynamic process of repression and the instinctual dynamic nature of the repressed. Defined as the cornerstone of psychoanalysis, repression was considered the major, if not the primary, cause of psychic distress. The analytic method sought to undo repression, the enemy of health, happiness and achievement. Analogies, therefore, between analyst and surgeon were not inappropriate to a struggle with unknown forces hidden within the unsuspecting mind of the consciously hopeful and co-operative patient. The positive relationship which Freud suggested would develop spontaneously, in the absence of serious errors, was necessary in the opening stages of treatment. 'The patient . . . must have formed a sufficient attachment (transference) to the physician for his emotional relationship to him to make a fresh flight impossible' (1910, p. 226). Once established, this relationship represented an acceptable, primarily conscious component of transference which would, on the whole, take care of itself.

This formulation, as Freud hints, was appropriate at a time which antedated psychoanalysis as a comprehensive theory of mental development, structure and function. As early as 1904, Freud nevertheless clearly distinguished between neurosis and the character of the patient who developed neurotic symptoms. He spelled out, in some detail, certain character attributes necessary for successful psychoanalytic work. He did not, however, initially ascribe these positive qualities to specific developmental phases. Nor did he discuss the problems relevant to the establishment of this basic relationship, which could be just as great a barrier to successful analysis as intense transference resistance or disturbing countertransference on the part of the analyst.

The structural approach led to modifications in the hypothetical model and inevitable changes in the theory of the therapeutic process. The analyst was subsequently defined in terms of his position *vis-à-vis* ego, superego and id. As a superego surrogate, he mitigated the harsh severity of the neurotic superego (Strachey, 1934). Since Richard Sterba's 1934 paper, the analyst's alliance with the healthy part of the patient's ego which had made a 'therapeutic split' has been increasingly emphasized. Freud himself defined the essence of the analytic situation: 'The analytic situation consists in our allying ourselves with the ego of the person under treatment, in order to subdue portions of his id which are uncontrolled—that is to say to include them in the synthesis of his ego' (1937, p. 235).

It is noteworthy that Freud here indicates that the analyst, i.e. a person, is one partner in this alliance. It is not, however, the patient but rather his ego which is described as the other partner. The analytic situation, like the analytic process, is thus defined in terms which primarily relate to the structure and function of the patient's individual psychic apparatus. This may be descriptively valid in many ways. It does not, however, explain the underlying meaning of the affective bond and the expectant faith which I believe implies a basic relationship between two persons—not egos.

In summary, neither Freud nor the other pioneer analysts bypassed the doctor–patient relationship as a necessary prerequisite to successful transference analysis. Like Freud, however, most contributors regarded the relationship either as an essentially stable, silent background which could take care of itself, or primarily as a feature of the opening stages of analysis. Edward Bibring made one of the most explicit and suggestive statements on this subject in his 1937 paper:

> In my opinion the analyst's attitude, and the analytical atmosphere which he creates, are fundamentally a reality-correction which adjusts the patient's anxieties about loss of love and punishment, the origin of which lies in childhood. Even if these anxieties later undergo analytical resolution I still believe that the patient's relationship to the analyst from which a sense of security emanates is not only a pre-condition of the procedure but also effects an immediate (apart from an analytical) consolidation of his sense of security which he has not successfully acquired or consolidated in childhood. Such an immediate consolidation—which, in itself, lies outside the field of

analytic therapy—is, of course, only of permanent value if it goes along with the co-ordinated operation of analytic treatment (1937, pp. 182–3).

This statement merits discussion for several reasons; first, the basic necessity of a secure relationship between patient and analyst is clearly acknowledged; second, its value is attributed to alleviation of primitive anxieties about loss of love and punishment; yet third, and most important, this 'consolidation' or alleviation is explicitly defined as being 'outside the field of analytic therapy'. This last statement must be understood within its historical context. Bibring (1937) and Sterba (1934), as well as other analysts doing pioneer ego analysis, attributed therapeutic alliance to available mature ego functions. They described the process of therapy mainly in terms of intrapsychic systems. An object relationship coloured by early anxieties, however essential, was almost by definition excluded from any active role in the analytic process. Melanie Klein and her school had taken a very different approach to the significance of early object relations. Introjection, projection, and primitive anxieties relevant to loss and retribution were regarded as pervasive. Transference as an object relationship involved revival in a new setting of the earliest conflicts. Failure in infancy to master the depressive position not only impaired later object relations and definitive ego functions, but also determined anxieties such as those described by Bibring in the opening phases of analysis. These anxieties, moreover, continue to dominate the analytic situation to such a degree that little, if any, distinction is clearly elaborated between transference as therapeutic alliance, and the transference neurosis as a manifestation of resistance.

It is not my purpose in this chapter to enter controversial areas in respect of the bearing of psychic events, occurring in the earliest days of life, on the analytic situation. Let us rather note the analogies between Freud's 'expectant faith' (1905*a*), Bibring's reference to early objective anxieties (1937), Erikson's 'basic trust' (1950) and Klein's mastery of the depressive position (1948). Each of these clearly refers to object relationships which derive from relatively early experience. Each of them also implies sufficient psychic development to include self-object differentiation, and a capacity for positive trusting object relationships and/or their converse. Each of them, finally, implies with greater or lesser specificity the potential vulnerability of such relationships to frustration, danger, separation or loss. The analytic situation not only involves all these, but also includes, as an inevitable concomitant, regression.

In Chapter 10, originally presented at the 19th Congress of the I.P.A. in 1955, certain controversial approaches to the significance and interpretation of regression were summarized. At that time the term 'therapeutic alliance' was introduced in relation to then current knowledge. A number of contributions have subsequently been made in which the primitive features of the analytic situation have been approached. Phyllis Greenacre (1958), Hans Loewald (1960), René Spitz (1956) and Maxwell Gitelson (1962) have placed considerable emphasis on certain aspects which in many ways comprise a repetition of the early mother–child relationship. Greenacre has in this context spoken of the 'matrix' of transference. Gitelson, in his paper 'The Curative Factors in Psychoanalysis' (1962), utilized a term introduced by Spitz who had spoken of the 'diatrophic function' of the analyst—his healing intention to 'maintain and support' the patient. Leo Stone (1961) has well summarized this aspect of psychoanalysis in his monograph *The Psychoanalytic Situation.*

The basic question which remains controversial concerns the significance of this primitive aspect of the relationship to the analyst in promoting or impeding analytic progress towards a maturational goal. Freud (1937) and Bibring (1937), for example, regard the establishment of rapport and the alleviation of early objective anxiety as a necessary but essentially extra-analytic prerequisite. Once established, they appear to imply that it is the mature ego of the patient which becomes the active partner in therapeutic alliance. Klein and her followers, in contrast, noting the infantile source of manifest anxiety in the opening stages of analysis, regard this anxiety as the major area of transference interpretation. The related Kleinian tendency to make little technical differentiation between interpretation at levels more primitive than the depressive position and those which, as Bibring implies, consolidate optimal early achievements, highlights controversy, and minimizes areas of potential agreement. Conversely, however, emphasis on the mature ego as the partner in therapeutic alliance, to the relative exclusion from the analytic process of primitive objective anxiety, needs amendment in the light of our current state of knowledge.

The impact of early object relations on basic ego functions is no longer open to serious question. In this context, it is the major thesis of this chapter that certain basic features of definitive psychic structure depend on qualitative aspects of early experience and on the nature of the first definitive ego identifications. It must be emphasized that the basic ego functions essential for later maturation, including the capacity for therapeutic alliance, develop during a period when the child is still relatively helpless and necessarily dependent on others. These basic functions concern the capacity to maintain basic trust in the absence of immediate gratification, the capacity to maintain self-object differentiation in the absence (relative or absolute) of the needed object, and the potential capacity to accept realistic limitations.

It may be suggested that no patient is so mature or so stable in respect of these capacities that the analytic situation fails to elicit some primitive objective anxiety which may be differentiated from the specific content of the transference neurosis. The degree and quality of such anxiety in the opening stages of psychoanalysis are subject to considerable variation. The patient's whole life experience, including the events which have preceded the commencement of analysis, will obviously play an important role. In essence, however, the initial stage involves achievement of a special object relationship which determines the nature, quality and stability of therapeutic alliance, which may thus be defined as both an object relationship and an ego identification.

This, I believe, implies more than the extra-analytic alleviation of objective anxiety which Bibring (1937) described so perceptively. It applies to the analytic situation, the concept of inseparability of object relations from ego attributes, which has become more and more prominent in recent studies of early infantile development. In Chapter 7 I concluded: 'It may prove that psychoanalytic truth cannot be adequately expressed in abstract terms based on the individual psychic apparatus.' As already indicated, discussions of the analytic process, like many theoretical reconstructions of early development, have focused primarily on events occurring within the individual psychic apparatus. It is proving increasingly difficult to understand individual development without a full consideration of early object relationships. So too, it may be suggested, neither the analytic situation nor the analytic process may adequately be understood or described solely as an individual event. Both analyst and patient are active partners in a relationship, the nature and meaning of which constitute the essence of the analytic situation.

Of special interest to this subject is the work of Ernst Kris and those (e.g. Ritvo and Solnit, 1958) who have followed his fruitful suggestions regarding the influence of the mother's spontaneous adaptation to the child's innate potentialities, on the nature and stability of early ego identifications. In so far as the mother responds intuitively and without ambivalence during the period ante-dating self-object differentiation, the child will have optimal opportunities to internalize and integrate an essentially positive ego identification. If, however, the mother is seriously rigid, withdrawn or ambivalent, the ego identification will be less secure, self-esteem unsatisfactory, and the capacity for basic trust impaired. Since no mother is perfect and since, in addition, innumerable variables are involved, the basic ego qualities already noted must be repeatedly reintegrated, via old or new object relations, when they are threatened by stress or regression. Such reintegration, particularly in the opening phases of analysis, not only re-establishes past achievements but also initiates the further ego growth and maturation which will reach its culmination in the terminal stages of the psychoanalytic process.

The nature and degree of active intervention on the part of the analyst in the opening hours of analysis have been a matter of considerable discussion and controversy. In particular, there is significant difference of opinion as to what may be defined as transference interpretation in this initial phase. There is a very general agreement to the effect that the transference neurosis usually develops gradually and that premature interpretations may therefore have untoward effects. This general position has, however, tended in certain respects to encourage prolonged silence, lack of participation, and a somewhat rigid attitude, particularly in the initial experience of candidates in training. The conviction has become somewhat widespread that, in the opening hours, any reference to the analytic situation or to the person of the analyst constitutes a transference interpretation of a type to be avoided. In contrast, it is my increasing conviction, particularly in respect of the supervised treatment of analysable neurotic patients, that serious problems in subsequent transference analysis may frequently be attributed to failure in the initial phases of treatment to achieve a secure therapeutic alliance by suitable verbal intervention. Clinical examples to illustrate this statement have been presented in Chapter 11.

Ernst Kris related the concept of early ego identification to that of the mother's adaptation to the child's innate potentialities. The position of the analyst in the opening phases of treatment must here be compared and contrasted. I am suggesting neither that the analytic patient resembles a newborn infant nor that the analyst's role is explicitly maternal. I am, however, proposing that from the outset the analytic situation demands from the patient maximal mobilization of ego characteristics which in large part depend on the success achieved at a relatively early stage of psychic development. Such mobilization will be fostered by intuitive adaptive responses on the part of the analyst which may well be compared to those of the successful parent. In the opening phases, however, the analyst is not responding to predominantly innate potentialities which originally preceded self-object differentiation. He is rather responding to anxieties aroused by threatened impairment of previous more or less solid achievement. Though regression is an inevitable concomitant of the analytic process, it must be contained. The patient must retain and reinforce his capacity for basic trust and positive ego identification in order to facilitate the analytic process which depends on regression, potentially in the service of the ego. I believe that what I am saying here constitutes one of the crucial differences between my point of view and that of the Kleinian analysts.

In so far as a patient begins analysis when he is already in a stage of threatened or partial ego regression, the analytic process cannot be initiated until the basic ego capacities prerequisite to genuine insight and affective learning have been re-established. This immediate goal requires a new positive object relationship which at first may be described in terms of Bibring's consolidation. In brief, the analyst helps the patient to recover, at least in the analytic relationship, the ego capacities which have previously been adequate in areas outside the sphere of neurotic conflict, i.e. Heinz Hartmann's (1939) conflict-free and/or autonomous ego functions utilizing neutralized ego-syntonic instinctual energy. The decision, it may be added, as to whether individual patients may be recommended for personal analysis depends primarily on positive evidence during initial evaluation that these essential ego resources are potentially available.

These positive ego attributes are often temporarily impaired in analysable patients by anxiety, depression or the instinctual regression characteristic of neurotic symptom formation. They are also readily threatened by the anxiety mobilized in many patients as a consequence of the technical demands of traditional analysis. Absence of this type of anxiety need not imply greater maturity, a better capacity for therapeutic alliance, or a speedier development of the transference neurosis. It is, in fact, all too frequently encountered in character neurosis, particularly counterphobic and obsessional, in highly intellectualized candidates, and in others for whom a personal analysis is a consciously desired source of added self-esteem. In such patients it may take some time for the analysis to 'get off the ground'. The first significant signs of genuine analytic work will usually be accompanied by manifest anxiety which relates more to problems in establishing therapeutic alliance, i.e. the analytic situation, than it does to reported material which is expressed in terms of transference neurosis.

In so far, therefore, as the achievement of therapeutic alliance represents a remobilization of preanalytic positive resources, it is to be regarded as an essential prerequisite rather than an integral feature of the analytic process itself. From this point of view, Bibring's formulation remains valid. It should also be noted that a similar goal may represent a major feature in the psychotherapy of maturational or situational crises and the long-term treatment of seriously disturbed patients. However, the specific features of psychoanalysis differentiate the analytic situation from the related tasks which, as Freud himself acknowledged, characterize the doctor–patient relationship in every therapeutic endeavour.

These specific features, though familiar to us all, nevertheless bear repetition in the context of their impact on the basic ego capacities already noted. The analytic patient must place himself in a passive, recumbent position. He must abandon certain controls which have determined both the form and content of his verbal communiations. He must relinquish the regular feedback, verbal and perceptual, which he can ordinarily anticipate. He must accept, in good faith, certain rules of procedure which he may not genuinely comprehend. To fulfil these demands it is necessary that both the goal of the analysis, as well as the other participant, the analyst, should be of central importance to the patient, who must at the same time recognize and accept the fact that the relationship is not equally reciprocal. He must therefore tolerate the anxiety, helplessness, and loss of self-esteem this situation easily arouses. He is asked, nevertheless, to have confidence in an unseen, often silent companion in this new and strange enterprise, to separate his wishes from his needs and, finally, to establish the new relationship and the new identification which will change his own orientation towards himself.

The demands of the analytic situation in many ways parallel the earlier experiences in which the basic ego capacities already noted were originally established. It is hardly surprising that, whether or not the patient had been in distress before, his relative success or failure in these basic developmental tasks is inevitably subject to stress as the relationship develops. Therapeutic alliance in the analytic situation does not therefore represent a simple consolidation of previous achievements in a setting fostering current adaptation. Rather it demands mobilization and maintenance of certain basic ego attributes in a situation which also involves the relative sacrifice of others. The analytic patient must retain maximal basic trust; he must contain both anxiety and depressive affect. His reality testing must remain intact. At the same time he is asked to relinquish crucial inner defences and controls against ego-alien impulses and fantasies previously motivated by signals of internal danger. This involves far more than extra-analytic consolidation of primitive anxiety. Though certain of its general features may be seen in other circumstances, it is primarily in the analytic situation that regression involving emergence of primitive, aggressive and erotic fantasies is fostered in a setting which also demands utilization and reinforcement of the complex, mature ego capacities integral to genuine psychological insight.

In discussing the analytic situation I have focused on the

difficulties inherent in a formulation of therapeutic psychoanalysis as an individual event. Both analyst and patient are active partners in a relationship, the nature and meaning of which constitute the essence of the analytic situation. The goal of individual therapeutic analysis primarily concerns the growth of one partner in the analytic situation; namely, the patient. The successful analyst, though he too may profit, does not change substantially during any one analysis in respect of his own mental structure or function, his basic attitude to the patient or his goal: successful analytic resolution of the patient's problems. Such changes, both favourable and unfavourable, do of course occur. However, I will assume the hypothetical ideal of and analysis unmodified by undesirable countertransference reactions, focusing primarily on the nature of the progressive changes which take place within the psychic apparatus of the patient. The analyst's role, both explicit and implicit, may in this context be examined as part of the patient's perceptual experience.

There are, of course, wide variations in the individual style of the analyst, whatever his orientation. In addition I have already referred to substantial controversy as to the relative accessibility of unconscious instinctual derivatives and the unconscious defences against their emergence. Such disagreement derives from differences in our theories of mental development, structure and function. They are reflected in our technique of clinical psychoanalysis. How far and in what way the analyst's silence or interpretative activity fosters or impedes the analytic process presents a central area of continued controversy.

Traditional analysts emphasize the strength, the automatic nature, and above all the degree to which the ego's defences are genuinely unconscious at the beginning of analysis. This theoretical position is reflected in the analyst's inactivity during the opening stages of treatment. Such inactivity may elicit anxiety, anger and/or depression. It may also impose a considerable degree of sensory deprivation. This, we have come to know, tends to foster regression. The transference neurosis in its classical form is the result of formal, topographical and temporal regression. Like dreams, symptom formation and other regressive states, instinctual derivatives which are labile and fluid partially replace previously automatic defences. Unless specific transference fantasies are expressed, the traditional psychoanalyst confines his intervention to the minimum consistent with a sustained therapeutic alliance.

In contrast, analysts of the Kleinian school believe that primitive fantasy is directed towards the analyst at the commencement of treatment. Implicitly, they stress the primitive features of the level of development which few of us can reach unless we have the benefit of analysis. Transference material is not mainly attributed to a regressive process, the emergence of which requires time, patience and analytic inactivity. Early fantasy, early anxiety, and the more labile defences against instinct such as projection, introjection, and projective identification may be verbalized in the transference as soon as analysis begins. Such material, though it may be regarded as 'deep' in the sense that it derives from a primitive, archaic level, is believed to be accessible to direct interpretation. The ego's automatic, unconscious defences against anxiety and depression are not thus regarded as significant barriers to early transference interpretation.

The theories underlying the persistent and continuing dichotomy between those who advocate early and continuous transference interpretation and those who, in contrast, emphasize the barriers imposed by the ego's defences were epitomized in the two papers already mentioned by Richard Sterba and James Strachey. Sterba, as already noted, referred to the maturity of that part of the ego which allies itself with the analyst during the analytic process. The object relationship implicit in ego identification with the analyst received relatively little emphasis. Sterba nevertheless clearly recognized both the reality of the analyst and the relation of the ego's therapeutic split to early superego formation.

Strachey's theory of psychic development and the therapeutic process was significantly influenced by Kleinian psychology. He concentrated, for example, on the archaic primitive fantasies released in the course of transference analysis. This is compatible with the contemporary Kleinian hypothesis that the primitive and archaic are readily accessible to transference interpretation. Strachey attributes the emergence of such material to the analyst's role as an auxiliary superego, more permissive than the unconscious, archaic superego of the patient. Such a formulation does not necessarily imply that regression is prerequisite to the emergence of the transference neurosis. The patient's realistic perception of the analyst is nevertheless regarded as an essential concomitant of the analytic process.

It may be proposed that Strachey's discussion of the therapeutic process refers to a period after which the analytic situation has been established and integrated. His presentation may thus be compared and contrasted with traditional formulations regarding the interpretation of the transference neurosis. Therapeutic changes, according to Strachey, are attributable to those interpretations which he defined as 'mutative'. These, according to his description, have two separate stages. In the first the patient becomes conscious of a small quantity of id energy, that is, primitive fantasy. Strachey goes on to say:

> Since the analyst is . . . the *object* of the patient's id-impulses, the quantity of these impulses which is now released into consciousness will become consciously directed towards the analyst. This is the critical point. If all goes well, the patient's ego will become aware of the contrast between the aggressive character of his feelings and the real nature of the analyst. . . . The patient, that is to say, will become aware of a distinction between his archaic phantasy object and the real external object (1934, pp. 142–3).

Although stated in different terminology, Strachey's emphasis on the reality of the analyst as essential to a successful mutative interpretation is largely compatible with many recent contributions. Greenson, Stone, Gitelson, Greenacre and others have emphasized the reality of the doctor–patient relationship as an essential feature of successful analysis. Our differences concern the role of regression in the release of transference fantasy. It is easy to understand that those analysts who regard the primitive as readily accessible place relatively little emphasis on the regressive components of successful transference interpretation. Such analysts recognize few contraindictions to early and continuous transference interpretation. In traditional theory the transference neurosis is considered contingent on regression and the concomitant modification of unconscious defences. The analyst who accepts this orientation regards silence and inactivity as an essential factor in promoting such regression. The analyst's activity, however appropriate, tends to counteract regression by its sensory impact. This, as already noted, is necessary if serious regression appears to be imminent. In general, however, the position is maintained that continued interpretative activity tends to interfere with the emergence of an analysable transference neurosis.

According to this point of view the emergence of a transference neurosis is contingent on the regressive modification of neurotic defences. According to Strachey, however, the release of primitive fantasy is implicitly progressive. It is determined by the patient's perception of the analyst as a less threatening person than the internalized parental objects. Id derivatives are kept out of consciousness by the archaic superego which substantially influences the patient's perception of reality. As the patient internalizes a new, less punitive superego, unconscious primitive content is more readily released. In so far as the patient passes the critical point of reality testing, unconscious barriers to maturation imposed by the superego have been substantially removed. Both symptom formation and the transference neurosis are thus mainly attributed to the conflicts and fantasies which arise during the early months of life. Since oedipal fantasies arise during a period when aggression is more powerful than libidinal genital positive wishes, the negative components of the oedipal triangle are far more attributable to primitive instinct than to a realistic conflict which involves three individuals. This theory makes it difficult clearly to distinguish between hostility which derives from the most primitive sources and feelings of rivalry towards a known and loved object.

One effect of basic theories on our clinical understanding revolves on the significance of regression during analysis. To quote Strachey's summary:

> The final result of psycho-analytic therapy is to enable the neurotic patient's whole mental organization, which is held in check at an infantile stage of development, to continue its progress towards a normal adult state. The principal effective alteration consists in a profound qualitative modification of the patient's super-ego, from which the other alterations follow in the main automatically (1934, p. 159).

We would all agree with part of this statement, i.e. in our hope that our successfully analysed patients will 'progress towards a normal adult state'. One major difference concerns our understanding of what is meant by 'an infantile stage of development'. Another concerns the concept of automatic progress.

Many contemporary analysts emphasize the continued impact throughout life of the experiences which determine the quality and stability of early object relations. A secure one-to-one relationship must be established, maintained, and continuously reintegrated during the course of therapeutic analysis. The major conflicts, however, which determine the definitive ego defences of analysable neurotics did not occur in a one-to-one relationship. Though they may have retreated, they reached in childhood a developmental level at which a genuine triangular oedipal conflict had at least begun to emerge. The childhood resolution of this conflict, whether healthy or pathological, results in the establishment of a relatively closed system in respect of certain id derivatives. Backward movement, i.e. regression, which reopens the conflict is thus regarded as a necessary preliminary to the progressive mastery which is a common goal of all analysts, whatever their frame of reference.

The area of classical transference analysis thus involves reopening those conflicts which had previously been dealt with by neurotic, excessive or inadequate defences in an attempt to achieve a more adaptive resolution. This, however, is only possible if the basic ego functions which remain contingent on secure object relations are not only maintained but progressively strengthened. Psychoanalysis may well be compared in complexity for both patient and analyst to the infantile neurosis for both child and parent. The analyst's role is not confined to interpretation of the transference neurosis. He must remain objective and maintain adequate distance in interpretation of fantasies and wishes derived from the repressed, forgotten past. In this role he resembles the parent who can recognize, without gratifying, the derivatives of the child's incestuous fantasies during the infantile neurosis. At the same time, he must ally himself with the patient, remaining an object for continued positive ego identification. Of special importance in this context is the continual mutual recognition that passive acceptance of the inevitable is just as basic to psychic maturity as are active responses and adaptive mastery in available areas of gratification and achievement.

I am thus proposing a dual approach to the therapeutic process in psychoanalysis. This, I believe, highlights the intimate relationship between the analytic situation and the analytic process. The analyst must continue throughout to respond intuitively to affect, indicating the patient's basic need to feel accepted and understood as a real person. He must, at the same time, objectively recognize and interpret verbalizations and non-verbal behaviour which reveal wishes and fantasies derived from the transference neurosis proper. Here the analyst serves primarily as the displaced object of unresolved, unconscious infantile conflict. Successful analysis thus demands, at all times, recognition of the difference between the transference neurosis which is subject to infinite changeability, and the core of therapeutic alliance which, like other basic ego identifications, retains a continuous stable nucleus.

It must be recognized, however, that the basic identifications originally internalized in pregenital dyadic object relations are subject to both positive and negative modification during the emergence, working through, and passing of the triangular conflict which characterizes the infantile neurosis. During this period the child initiates what will later become his definitive sexualized identity. His perception of internal danger will mobilize intrapsychic defences against ego-alien instinctual impulses. These defences, among which repression and related mechanisms are dominant in the future neurotic, may also impair to a greater or lesser extent the basic self-esteem which had originally been initiated.

A major goal during the opening stages of analysis may be defined as reintegrating as far as possible previously achieved developmental tasks, with particular reference to self-esteem and other basic ego attributes. This is prerequisite to the regression ultimately in the service of adaptation and mastery which characterizes an analysable transference neurosis. The analytic process may then be understood as a modified repetition of the working through and resolution of the infantile neurosis. It not only changes the perception of internal danger and the need to respond with those automatic unconscious defences which may be defined as excessive or neurotic. It also results in progressive modification of those identifications internalized during this same period which had previously contributed to neurotic character traits or symptom formation. As this takes place there are changes in the content of the transference material and concurrent progress in respect of the maturity and the stability of the therapeutic alliance. (For clinical illustrations, see Chapter 11.)

Termination of a successful analysis leads to essential autonomy and independence. As the end approaches, however, residual passive, dependent wishes are inevitably revived and reinforced. (For a clinical illustration, see Chapter 6.) The analyst's position during this period should be distinguished from his attitude during the earlier stages of treatment. He is no longer in a position comparable to that of a parent who responds to the passive regressive components of the infantile neurosis. He might better be compared to a parent willing and able to foster the maturation and autonomy of his children during late adolescence and early maturity. In other words, the degree of passivity essential to the analytic process represents an essentially ego-alien infantile wish during the period of termination. The patient must now achieve a mature acceptance of realistic limits, combined with active mobilization of autonomy and independence. The analyst, like the good parent, is retained as an object for continued positive ego identification. In addition, the analyst, again like the parent, remains a potentially available object in case of future need. No child or patient achieves emotional maturity until he accepts the fact that he is not so invulnerable that if need arose he would not feel free to return for advice or help.

In conclusion, psychoanalytic treatment presents many analogies to the early developmental process. In regard to both I have amplified the dual approach introduced in Chapter 11. I have thus differentiated between that which is involved in the establishment and maintenance of object relations and ego identifications from that which is contained within the psychic apparatus of the individual as a result of defensive mechanisms mobilized by signal anxiety. The former relates to an essentially open system which involves the continued integration of new identifications in the setting of positive object relations. The latter concerns ego-alien wishes, fantasies and related memories in a relatively closed system. Successful development in the later stages of childhood is contingent upon the maintenance of basic object relationships achieved in the initial stages. The qualities in the analyst which concern the analytic situation correspond in many ways to the qualities which help a good parent to foster the child's development towards maturity and independence. Psychic development, however, involves both progressive and regressive manifestations at all times. Such regression can only lead to active mastery when basic ego functions are maintained and strengthened. This statement applies to the infantile neurosis, adolescence and other developmental crises. It is central to the developmental implications of controlled regression within the analytic situation.

13

AN OBSESSIONAL NEUROTIC: FREUD'S RAT MAN[1]

(1966)

This chapter is a re-examination of the first and possibly most famous obsessional patient discussed in detail by Sigmund Freud. It was my intention when I first undertook this study to base my discussion primarily on the 1909 report published in Freud's *Collected Papers.* Fortunately, however, I decided to re-read the case history in the *Standard Edition.* I was surprised and excited by the discovery I made—namely, the unique salvage of Freud's daily notes covering the first four months of this analysis. These informal notes, as James Strachey suggests, permit us to participate in Freud's continuous scrutiny of the material presented by his patient; in his awareness of areas in which the patient's conflicts may have impinged on his own; and in his concurrent reflections as to the possible significance of this analysis for more general understanding of the obsessional neurosis. His frank allusions, finally, to his own activity serve as salutary reminders of the degree to which the papers in which Freud recommended coldness, neutrality, and mirror-like detachment were based on an implicit differentiation between the analyst's position *vis-à-vis* the transference neurosis and the man's warm and spontaneous participation in the one-to-one doctor–patient relationship which is an indispensable feature of the analytic situation.

The 1909 publication provided concrete empirical material to demonstrate the continued impact of early instinctual life in determining the content and nature of adult symptomatology. It defined and elaborated in relation to this patient's thought processes most of the mechanisms which characterize the obsessional neurosis: reaction formation, indecision, isolation, un-

[1] Paper read at the 24th Congress of the International Psycho-Analytical Association, Amsterdam, in July 1965. First published in the *Int. J. Psycho-Anal.* (1966), **47**.

doing, intellectualization, and magical thinking. Despite the emphasis given to oedipal content in Freud's explicit interpretations, the anal sadistic implications of the patient's basic conflict were also clearly recognized. The regressive reemergence of unconscious, unresolved conflicts in both symptom formation and transference analysis were convincingly demonstrated. Last, but by no means least, Freud's repeated reference to the patient's positive attributes highlights one of the major criteria for analysability—namely, availability of the healthy, intact part of the patient's personality as one partner in the analytic situation.

In his introduction to the familiar 'Notes upon a Case of Obsessional Neurosis' (1909*a*) Freud described this patient's obsessional neurosis as one of moderate severity. The evaluation was made after the patient's analysis had been successfully completed. His symptoms, however (as described in the early phases of treatment), had at times been quite disabling. The possibility must therefore be entertained that Freud's evaluation was in part determined by his sensitivity to a conceptual distinction he was to make only two years later in 'Formulations on the Two Principles of Mental Functioning' (1911), a distinction between pathology determined by developmental failure of the ego and symptomatology attributable to instinctual fixation or regression.

Freud also acknowledged in the same introduction his drastic curtailment of this case and its treatment. The original notes suggest that the Rat Man, like Irma, moved in circles which impinged on Freud's social life, and that one reason for many of the omissions was protection of the patient's anonymity. Would Freud, however, have saved these notes if all his omissions had served their purpose? Surely this would have been an excellent reason for destroying them. He himself hinted at another explanation: 'I must confess that I have not yet succeeded in completely penetrating the complicated texture of a *severe* case of obsessional neurosis . . . an obsessional neurosis is in itself not an easy thing to understand—much less so than a case of hysteria' (1909*a*, p. 156).

Only four years later, in his paper on 'The Disposition to Obsessional Neurosis' (1913*b*), Freud himself indicated the degree to which both obsessional and hysterical symptomatology might prove highly deceptive. The criteria for analysability are not determined by the content or the severity of the presenting symptoms. As Robert Knight (1953) has demonstrated, obsessional thinking and compulsive behaviour may serve as bulwarks, however unsatisfactory, behind which psychotic disorder remains partially hidden. It may be suggested, therefore, that the obsessional patients whom Freud described as either severe or not yet understood may have differed from the Rat Man with respect to basic ego functions. The Wolf Man (1918) comes to mind as a case in point. Mark Kanzer (1952) has emphasized the acting out element in this patient's behaviour during critical stages of his analysis. I would propose, rather, that this same behaviour, which after all occurred before the sanctification of the couch, illustrated in dramatic form those ego attributes which are prerequisite to the crucial therapeutic split between fantasy or transference and reality or therapeutic alliance. The Rat Man, it will be recalled, remained at all times aware of and disturbed by the ego-alien negative transference fantasies which determined his behaviour. In addition, despite his intellectual defences, his tendency to isolate and his use of denial, the Rat Man demonstrated in his dreams, fantasies and associations the capacity for instinctual regression which is a necessary concomitant of an analysable transference neurosis.

In the original publication, successful though it was in demonstrating both the form and the content of obsessional symptoms, some of Freud's theoretical speculations remained difficult and obscure. This is particularly striking in his efforts to account for the inexorable either–or which characterized the alternating feelings of love and hate which the Rat Man directed towards his father and his lady:

> The conflicts of feeling in our patient which we have here enumerated separately were not independent of each other, but were bound together in pairs. His hatred of his lady was inevitably coupled with his attachment to his father, and inversely his hatred of his father with his attachment to his lady. But [and this is the statement I wish to emphasize] the two conflicts of feeling which result from this simplification—namely, the opposition between his relation to his father and to his lady, and the contradiction between his love and his hatred within each of these relations—had no connection whatever

with each other, either in their content or in their origin (1909*a*, p. 238).

Freud's reference to this 'either–or' is worthy of comment, as is his discussion of sharp differentiation, on the one hand, between the dichotomy masculine–feminine and, on the other, the love–hate conflict within individual object relations. It might be suggested that his discussion of these problems could well be compared with his own references to the obscure and puzzling features of those dream elements which impinge most closely on problems of decisive and crucial importance. Freud himself presented a hypothesis for the occurrence of 'such a strange state of affairs' (which might aptly be cited by a follower of Melanie Klein or Donald Fairbairn): 'At a very early age, somewhere in the prehistoric period of infancy, the two opposites should have been split apart . . .'.

What is implicit in the discussion is a distinction (which could not have been made in 1909) between substantial failure to integrate perceptions and emotions initially experienced as mutually exclusive—e.g. pain and pleasure, love and hate, activity and passivity, omnipotence and helplessness, and regressive impairment during neurotic symptom formation of integrations which had previously been established. Recognition and substantial mastery of the conflict between love and hate which Freud described as 'a strange state of affairs' is familiar to us today as one of the crucial developmental tasks integral to healthy self-object differentiation and early ego identification. The developmental achievements which determine at least one of the criteria for analysability concern this specific area. The individual who, like the Rat Man, is capable of maintaining a real object relationship despite the emergence of conflicting negative feelings has been able, at whatever sacrifice, to recognize and tolerate concurrent feelings of love and hate towards one and the same object. His love, moreover, though perhaps by a narrow margin, has been substantially successful in achieving what might truly be described as a pyrrhic victory. In his case, the nature of this victory was shown by the crippling inhibitions, the shifting doubt, and the smoke cloud of compulsions which characterized his severe but nevertheless analysable obsessional neurosis. Despite the inexorable 'either–or' which characterized the alternation between love and hate in his neurotic symptom formation and transference neurosis, the Rat Man proved capable of tolerating considerable ambivalence in the analytic situation.

It is not surprising that Freud's brilliant speculations touched on the phase of psychic development in which this capacity is first initiated, namely, what was then the prehistoric period of early infancy. Neither the importance of early object relations nor their possible relevance to the analytic situation had been envisaged in 1909. Freud's then current theory of object relations was indicated by a long footnote in which he stressed the overriding importance of early autoerotism and instinctual gratification. It is well known, however, that the stages of ego development and significant object relations which intervene between autoerotic activity preceding self-object differentiation, and the capacity for adult heterosexual object love, still remain one of the most difficult and controversial areas in psychoanalytic theory.

Freud's reconstruction of the Rat Man's early development was inevitably based on his approach to instinctual impulses and autoerotic gratification. The father was seen as an important real object—one who interfered with or threatened his son's instinctual impulses. Early object love, either pregenital or genital, was given relatively little attention. The patient's mother, for example, was only mentioned in six brief, essentially unrevealing, statements. Although, in addition, Freud acknowledged the possible importance of the death of the patient's elder sister, he was led to the reconstruction that its primary significance related to the patient's subsequent conviction that 'you die if you masturbate'.

In striking contrast with the 1909 publication, there are more than forty references to a highly ambivalent mother–son relationship in the original clinical notes. Freud published his initial consultation almost verbatim with one significant omission: 'After I had told him my terms, he said he must consult his mother.' The patient, it will be recalled, was 29 years old at that time. On 18 October he reported that he had not taken over his inheritance from his father but had left it with his mother, who allowed him a small amount of pocket-money. Mention of his mother was relatively scanty during the first weeks of his analysis.

As the analytic situation became more secure, however, there is evidence to suggest an increasingly positive identification with Freud, who noted with some pleasure on 8 December: 'He has stood up manfully against his mother's lamentation over his having spent 30 florins of pocket-money during the last month instead of 16.' On 19 December his negative feelings about his mother became manifest and intense: 'He gets everything that is bad in his nature . . . from his mother's side. . . . He hands over all his money to his mother because he does not want to have anything from her.' These and many other references to financial problems, cleanliness and dirt, hostile fantasies and the reaction formations against them clearly point to a major area of instinctual fixation.

There are, in addition, notes which suggest that Freud perceived, although he did not conceptualize, the type of mother–child relationship and ego identification characteristic of many future obsessional characters and obsessional neurotics. On 21 December Freud says: 'He has been identifying himself with his mother in his behaviour and treatment-transferences. . . . It seems likely that he is also identifying himself with his mother in his criticisms of his father and is thus continuing the differences between his parents within himself.' Could we have a better description of the process later to be defined as introjection? Is there anywhere in our literature a more precise account of the mechanism Anna Freud was to describe as 'identification with the aggressor'? Longitudinal observations of young children have in recent years demonstrated the significance of this defensive identification as one important precursor of the harsh superego of the future obsessional.

It must be noted, however, that this highly ambivalent relationship with his mother was not expressed in the opening phases of the Rat Man's analysis. It only emerged after the patient had mastered some of his ambivalence and established a positive therapeutic alliance with his analyst. The fact that he could do so raises questions as to how far unresolved ambivalence and significant identification with the aggressor had characterized this patient's initial relationship with his mother.

Alternative hypotheses which might help us to understand his positive ego attributes may be suggested. First, that an essentially satisfactory infantile mother–child relationship had been threatened or impaired by the birth of a younger brother when he was 18 months old. Second, that he had turned during his second and third years to a sister older enough to have enjoyed a maternal role. Third, that his pre-oedipal relationship with a father, who emerges as an essentially warm and loving parent, had been predominantly positive. An essentially normal, although partially displaced, oedipal triangle may thus have emerged before the onset of this sister's fatal illness. Both his severe childhood neurosis and his adult predisposition to an obsessional illness might in this case be attributed to certain regressive responses to trauma rather than the continuation into adult life of initial developmental failure.

The original notes provide many hints of the importance of this relationship to both children. Katherine's attachment to the patient is indicated by her statement: 'On my soul, if you die I shall kill myself.' The patient reports a few recollections of Katherine's incipient illness. He remembers someone carrying her to bed; he remembers that she had for a long time complained of feeling tired. 'Once when Dr. P. was examining her he turned pale.' He also remembers asking, 'Where is Katherine?' and described his father sitting in a chair weeping. His famous —but not subjectively remembered—outburst of rage almost certainly occurred during the course of Katherine's fatal illness. In this affective storm the little boy attacked his father, calling him a 'towel', 'lamp' and 'plate'. Was this choice of inanimate objects determined, as Freud suggests, by the patient's lack of a wider vocabulary? Was it indicative of a direct death wish towards an oedipal rival? The separation from and impending loss of an important early object must also be considered. The outburst could be seen as representing in evidence his desperate longing for his sister. The terms of abuse might then have an additional meaning—reproach to a loved but devalued father for his withdrawal, unhappiness and inability to help or console the anguished child. Not only the sister, but also the father failed to meet the child's need for love and support.

I have elsewhere related similar acute affective responses to separation with the recognition and tolerance of depression as an ego state. Relative developmental failures in tolerating such unpleasant affect represent one important determinant of the ego defences which are predominant in the obsessional neurotic.

It may be noted that Berta Bornstein (1949) related the childhood neurosis of the future obsessional Frankie to his attempts to ward off depression during a period of separation from his mother. Neither the Rat Man nor Frankie appears to have acknowledged or demonstrated overt depression. The context within which the Rat Man's outburst of rage occurred suggests, however, that Katherine's illness and death may well have mobilized regressive defences against the re-emergence of depressive anxiety with its related feelings of helplessness. This may have involved subsequent reinforcement of the defences characteristic of the earlier anal sadistic developmental period—magical thinking, reaction formation, isolation, and intellectualization. It may also have led to substantial retreat from the triangular relations of the genital oedipal situation to the more primitive one-to-one relations of an earlier period. The 'either–or' which characterized his adult neurosis may thus have represented a revival in adult life of this earlier regressive response to trauma. The reported memory of childhood fears lest his parents could read his thoughts suggests, in addition, an incipient impairment of self-object differentiation and the use of projection as a mechanism of defence.

The early development of individuals who become healthy or analysable adults is characterized by the pregenital achievement of genuine one-to-one relations with both parents. In such circumstances the oedipal conflict can emerge and develop without sacrifice of sustained object relationships. Substantial developmental failure in the capacity for such object relations, although it may not preclude incestuous oedipal fantasies, usually involves an all or nothing quality which impairs the individual's capacity for a positive therapeutic alliance. Such developmental failure is to be differentiated from regressive responses to traumatic experience, which may sometimes present misleadingly similar symptomatology.

The loss of an incestuous object at a time when the attachment is intense may have long-term after-effects. In so far as the child experiences the loss as a punishment for his sexual wishes, his inhibitions, guilt and ambivalence would, as Freud indicated, be considerably increased. In addition, the ability to recognize and work through later bereavements may be seriously impaired as a result of early loss. Denial, a defence which should gradually diminish during healthy maturation, may be substantially reinforced.

The Rat Man's continued use of denial in adult life was conspicuous in his striking inability genuinely to recognize, grieve or accept the finality of his father's death. He failed, for example, to mention the fact that his father had been dead for nearly ten years when he first recounted the story of the rat punishment. Other episodes underlined his persistent feeling that his dead father might walk into the room. He frequently thought about him as though he were still alive. Although many of his fantasies in the area of sexual activity were overtly hostile, an undertone of sustained positive feeling is clearly apparent. The patient would have welcomed his father's return. His positive object relationship with his father appears to have been at least as important as the hostile oedipal rivalry which was stressed in the 1909 publication.

That Freud recognized the importance of the Rat Man's denial is indicated by his note of 23 December: 'I pointed out to him that this attempt to deny the reality of his father's death is the whole basis of his neurosis.' Freud is here obviously referring to his adult neurosis. I would like to suggest that a parallel but much earlier denial in respect of his sister Katherine had at least equal importance for the patient's predisposition. This, I believe, also determined his attachment in adult life to a young woman, Gisela, in whom he found a suitable replacement for his dead sister. From the published notes and daily record we get a picture of Gisela as (i) a first cousin; (ii) possibly too old for him (her age is not mentioned); (iii) almost certainly sterile, a fact which made her resemble a prepubertal little girl; and (iv) a woman who was subject to frequent serious and disabling periods of ill health. In addition, the fact that this cousin who was herself highly ambivalent may also have been 'abused' by her stepfather, and was at least as disturbed in respect of her psychosexual life as the patient, suggests that her own personality lent itself to a relationship characterized by many infantile features.

There is a wealth of material in the original notes to support the hypothesis that the Rat Man's persistent attachment to his ailing cousin represented an overdetermined, necessarily ambivalent effort to revive his sister as he last recalled her, namely, as an increasingly tired little girl who was finally carried away to the room in which she was to die. Recovery of this lost object entailed sacrifice—i.e. substantial renouncement of libidinal wishes. On 27 October he dreamt, in this context, that another sister was very ill. A friend told him: 'You can only save your sister by renouncing all sexual pleasure.' His cousin was not only sterile; she also suffered periods of illness during which it may be assumed that sexual interest was prohibited. During one such illness when 'he was most deeply concerned about her, there crossed his mind as he looked at her a wish that she might lie like that for ever'. Although the hostile death wishes which Freud deduced from this incident are not to be excluded, underlying fear of loss must also be acknowledged. In so far as Gisela represented Katherine, her illness may have been experienced as imminent death in the Rat Man's repressed unconscious.

It may be suggested that, just as Katherine's death had precipitated a childhood regression, his father's death, before he had reached full maturity, not only impeded adaptive utilization of a developmental second chance, but also undermined the precarious adjustment so far maintained. Neither loss, however, led to irreversible ego regression, as shown by his capacity to tolerate a difficult analytic situation. Some of the difficulties, it may be suggested, may have derived from his regressive wish to re-establish his passive pre-oedipal father–son relationship. Such wishes would inevitably conflict with oedipal rivalry and the unconscious search for the lost heterosexual object. These passive wishes may well have been an important factor in his inability to tolerate the couch and the defensively overdetermined negative transference material.

The analytic situation is a one-to-one relationship which draws on the strengths and reveals the weaknesses of the initial mastery of ambivalence in an essentially passive situation. The early mother–child relationship has been mentioned by many analysts. For example, Maxwell Gitelson (1962) made explicit reference to the importance of the analyst's diatrophic responses during the opening phases of clinical psychoanalysis. Phyllis Greenacre (1958) has referred to the 'matrix' of transference. I have in Chapter 15 attempted to delineate the parallels and the differences between the parents' empathic responses to a young child and the analyst's intuitive responses to his patient's affective needs.

It may be suggested that this patient's continued unresolved ambivalence towards his mother might have made him vulnerable to ego regression in an uncommunicative analytic situation. Freud's spontaneous responses, however, as reported during the first few months of the Rat Man's analysis, appear to have differed considerably from his later theoretical models—his communications were not limited to interpretation of the transference neurosis. He acknowledged his patient's anxiety and took him into his confidence. He praised and encouraged him. He corrected realistic misinformation and explained the analytic reasons why he could not allow the patient to withhold names. Despite the somewhat intellectualized terms in which some of both their verbalizations were phrased, the underlying atmosphere appears to have been one of mutual respect and considerable understanding. If, therefore, my hypothesis regarding the patient's early feelings towards his father is correct, his therapeutic alliance may have derived from his positive one-to-one relationship.

The original notes reveal Freud's comfort in correcting realistic misinformation and in other spontaneous interactions which might be regarded as questionable today. His subsequent recommendation of neutrality may have represented recognition of the fact that such interventions may sometimes prove unfortunate. Other patients may have responded less favourably to the type of activity which Freud showed in this analysis. The Rat Man's responses nevertheless illustrate a point which cannot be too strongly emphasized in our understanding of clinical psychoanalysis. A good analytic situation, although it may temporarily be distorted or modified, will not be undermined by occasional defections from traditional technique by the analyst. Conversely, if a good analytic situation has not been achieved, technically correct interpretations will have little, if any, therapeutic value.

Two brief examples will illustrate Freud's technique in this analysis. Someone had told the patient that a distant Hungarian relative of Freud's had been a criminal. The patient only reported this gossip after a painful struggle. Freud laughingly relieved the patient's anxiety, saying that he had no relatives in Budapest. Two days later the patient reported a more significant realistic reinforcement of his active negative transference neurosis. His sister had once remarked that Freud's brother Alex would be the right husband for the patient's lady. The patient's fear lest Freud had designs on him as a husband for his daughter was compounded by the fantasy that the patient's lady would be taken over by Freud's brother. The familiar hostile transference material was thus doubly determined. This example illustrates the realistic reasons for certain omissions; however, the patient's ability to report this disturbing gossip suggests that his response to the first correction had been helpful rather than harmful.

The second illustration is both startling and unusual. Freud's notes for 28 December commence as follows: 'He was hungry and was fed.' Direct responses to oral demands have sometimes been mentioned as an appropriate therapeutic concomitant to the treatment of psychotic patients. The indications for such procedures can be found in contemporary developmental theory concerning the genesis of psychosis. As already noted, however, Freud's 1909 understanding of psychic development placed little explicit emphasis on early maternal functions. While it is highly improbable that he regarded his action as a therapeutic manoeuvre, it is noteworthy that, just as the correction of misinformation had been followed on the earlier occasion by further revelations, the patient in this instance felt free to reject in words the gratification which he had partially accepted in fact. During the same hour he referred to his need to diet in order to lose weight. Within the next few days he verbalized with greater freedom the identification with his mother as an aggressor. He mentioned, in addition, that he had left the herring which had been offered untouched because he 'disliked herring intensely'. These responses suggest that an intervention which must be defined as unanalytic had not impeded the progress of this patient's treatment. The fact that he could reveal with increasing clarity his hostility to his mother, his comfort in rejecting part of the meal, verbalizing in this context certain criticisms of Freud, confirms the positive therapeutic alliance which he had achieved by the end of the year.

Neither the published report nor the original notes permit us fully to understand the significance of his symptomatic recovery. The report demonstrated both a positive therapeutic alliance and the emergence of an analysable transference neurosis. The original notes permit us to reconsider certain aspects of his childhood neurosis and adult predisposition within the context of contemporary theory. I would suggest that the little boy who grew up to be the Rat Man might not have developed a serious neurosis were it not for the impact of a significant loss sustained at the height of the infantile neurosis. His relatively brief psychoanalysis appears at the very least to have helped him to retrieve the developmental achievements which had been so undermined in early childhood. His positive identification with a father surrogate, Freud, may have been the central factor which impelled him towards greater mastery of unresolved intrapsychic conflict. The unresolved ambivalence surrounding his relationship with his mother may have remained a potential Achilles heel. He may, however, have become a well-integrated, somewhat obsessional character instead of a decompensated obsessional neurotic.

Although we have no final note as to the patient's definitive heterosexual achievement, it is nevertheless evident that Freud acted as an ally rather than a hostile menace in the patient's efforts to reintegrate genital potency and heterosexual object love. Whether and how far symptomatic remission would have enabled him (had he survived World War I) to reach and sustain his full potentiality must always remain an open question. Freud's willingness, however, to let him try his wings once his serious symptoms had disappeared is relevant to the recurrent problem as to the indications for interruption or termination of psychoanalysis. This patient might have been caught in an interminable analysis if theoretical considerations had taken precedence over the demands of reality.

14

THE SO-CALLED GOOD HYSTERIC[1]

(1968)

There was a little girl
And she had a little curl
Right in the middle of her forehead.
And when she was good
She was very, very good,
But when she was bad
She was horrid.

This nursery rhyme, familiar to most of us, is particularly applicable to the analysis of those female patients whose presenting symptomatology or character structure overtly suggests an unresolved genital oedipal situation. This leads to a presumptive diagnosis of hysteria, the condition which is still widely considered to be most responsive to traditional psychoanalysis. Kurt Eissler, for example, in discussing ego structure and analytic technique, suggested that hysteria can be taken as 'the baseline of the psychoanalytic therapy. . . . the earliest psychoanalytic model of hysteria pertains to an ego which has suffered that minimum of injury without which no neurosis would develop at all' (1953, p. 114).

J. O. Wisdom, in a more recent paper, however, asked a most pertinent question: 'Hysteria', he said, 'has been longest studied, and there is a feeling that more is known about it than about any other disorder. . . . Is this true? It seems to me on the contrary that there is much that is obscure about the theory of hysteria' (1961, p. 224).

My jingle alludes to one aspect of this obscurity, one which has been revealed by the very different responses to traditional

[1] Expanded from a paper read at the 25th Congress of the International Psycho-Analytical Association, Copenhagen, in July 1967. First published in the *Int. J. Psycho-Anal.* (1968), **49**.

analysis of patients initially diagnosed as hysterical. In a study based on a review of the first hundred patients evaluated for supervised analysis in Boston, a follow-up study was made of those patients who had been in treatment for more than a year. Those described as obsessional had all established a reasonably satisfactory analytic situation at the time we made our inquiry. None of them, however, had developed a clearly analysable, explicit transference neurosis. This finding is in keeping with Charles Rycroft's suggestion (cited by Wisdom, 1961) that the theory of primary process thinking might have been different if Freud had had a practice consisting mainly of obsessionals. Kurt Eissler makes a similar comment: 'Tentatively I would say that the discovery of psychoanalysis would have been greatly impeded, delayed, or even made impossible if in the second half of the nineteenth century the prevailing neurosis had not been hysteria' (1953, p. 114).

It is nevertheless generally recognized that most of the patients described in Freud's early studies were far more disturbed than patients currently referred to analysis who are diagnosed as hysterics. Despite careful screening, the results obtained with those patients originally described as hysterical and subsequently referred for supervised analysis were dramatically different from the reports submitted regarding obsessionals. As we have said, 'Our reports so far tend to indicate that hysterical patients are, to put it simply, very good or very bad patients' (Knapp *et al.*, 1960). The former had not only established a satisfactory analytic situation; they had also, in almost every case, developed a highly analysable transference neurosis after approximately one year of analysis. The latter, in contrast, may have developed an intense, highly sexualized transference neurosis, but with little evidence of a stable analytic situation. None of them appeared to have made any genuine progress towards analytic resolution of their presenting problems.

Wisdom's questioning of our understanding of hysteria is thus reflected by the very different responses of patients whose presenting symptoms appear to traditional psychoanalytic technique to be hysterical. He also noted that it was 'a matter of some astonishment to find that the sources in Freud for the syndrome and theory are scattered, unsystematic, strangely late, or non-existent' (1961, p. 236*n*). In a more recent paper entitled 'Hysterical Personality: A Re-evaluation', Barbara Easser and Stanley Lesser suggest that

> investigators such as the Boston Group have highlighted the need for greater diagnostic precision and evaluative formulation. . . . The terms hysteria, hysterical character, etc. are so loosely defined and applied so promiscuously that their application to diagnostic categories has become meaningless. The use of these labels for evaluation, analysability, or prognosis has become tantamount to predicting a throw of the dice (1965, p. 392).

This statement accords well with Eissler's attempt 'to demonstrate how little or how much a mechanism or a symptom as such may count, depending on the all-inclusive ego organization in which it occurs' (1953, p. 118). It is clear that neither hysterical symptomatology nor apparent hysterical character structure bears conclusive evidence to the relatively unmodified ego which can best respond to traditional psychoanalysis. Although Wisdom limits his theory to a discussion of male hysteria, he clearly reaches the conclusion that problems of ego identification must be taken into consideration. It is generally recognized that manifest hysterical symptomatology is, however, far more common in female than it is in male neurotics. It was partly for this reason that Easser and Lesser confined their discussion to female hysterics.

Although this statement is correct as far as manifest presenting symptomatology is concerned, it may nevertheless be somewhat misleading. Most typically, analysable men are likely to complain initially of problems which suggest an obsessional condition. Their overt symptoms more often relate to work than to heterosexual object relations. During the course of a successful analysis, however, most of these men clearly reveal evidence of an unresolved oedipal situation quite parallel to that shown by the most analysable hysterical women. Although, therefore, they could not be described as overtly hysterical, they nevertheless suffered from a mixed neurosis, with many hysterical features. In summary, the genesis of their adult neurosis proved in many ways to be comparable to the suggestions put forward in Chapter 13.

Easser and Lesser also excluded male patients for another reason: namely, their finding that in males, 'at least in Western society, hysteria is most often associated with effeminate characteristics' (1965, p. 393*n*). This finding is in keeping with the suggestion that the most analysable men are likely to utilize many obsessional defences. Such defences, although less pervasive, are also typically utilized by those hysterical women who have best responded to therapeutic analysis. In my own clinical experience male hysterics who have failed to mobilize adequate obsessional defences seldom belong to the most analysable group of male neurotics. At best, they belong to the group I will describe as 'potential good hysterics'. Frequently, however, their analysis reveals an underlying depressive character structure. At worst, they are as disturbed as the group of women I will describe as 'so-called good hysterics'. Usually, however, the male counterpart of this last group does not use transparent hysterical mechanisms. He falls rather more often into the group of so-called normal characters. These are the men whose deceptive external adaptation has been achieved with only minimal awareness of inner reality and with resultant marked defects in the area of affect tolerance.

Although my statements may have some significance for the treatment of male hysterics, this chapter really concerns female hysterics.

In my experience, women whose presenting symptomatology suggests a diagnosis of either hysterical character or hysterical symptomatology tend to fall into one of four subgroups, ranging from the most to the least analysable, depending on their response to therapeutic analysis. Of course, although each of these groups has clear distinguishing features in its most characteristic form, I do not wish to imply anything approaching rigid compartmentalization. The most analysable hysteric is vulnerable to regression in a bad analytic situation. Conversely, certain patients who have regressed before referral may initially present a clinical picture which suggests more serious disturbance than is actually the case.

My four groups may be briefly defined as follows:

First, there are 'true good hysterics', young women who are both prepared and ready for all aspects of traditional psychoanalysis.

Second, there are the 'potential good hysterics', young women whose development, symptomatology and character structure clearly suggest an analysable hysterical disorder. They are, however, less fully prepared or internally ready to make the serious commitment prerequisite to the establishment of a viable analytic situation.

Third, there are women with an underlying depressive character structure who frequently present manifest hysterical symptomatology to a degree which disguises their deeper pathology.

Fourth, there are women whose manifest hysterical symptomatology proves to be pseudo-oedipal and pseudo-genital. Such patients seldom meet the most important criteria for analysability.

This classification is based on a reconsideration of the relation between hysteria and the infantile oedipal situation. I am, in a manner of speaking, attempting to approach what Easser and Lesser described as an interesting paradoxical dissociation:

> On the one hand, the hysteric theoretically is considered to have achieved the highest libidinal level for neurotic fixation, i.e. phallic-oedipal, and on the other hand, the sufferers are regarded as frustrating, provocative, infantile, teasing, suggestible, irresponsible, non-intuitive, egocentric, non-productive citizens. As such they are regarded with contempt and disparagement (1965, pp. 391–2).

The paradox is, I believe, more apparent than real. It derives from a relative failure adequately to distinguish between instinctual progression and regression on the one hand, and the ego achievements prerequisite to the emergence, recognition and mastery of a genuine internal danger situation on the other. The story of Oedipus himself is not a good prototype for what we now mean by a potentially healthy infantile neurosis. His father was not a real person in relation to either Oedipus or his mother. He was a stranger by whom Oedipus had been abandoned. And Oedipus's mother, Jocasta, was in fact realistically available.

The myth nevertheless highlights the nature of the dilemma with which the child is most sharply confronted if and when he reaches a genuine oedipal conflict. It was not just fear that his father was stronger and might therefore castrate him which Freud emphasized in his discussion of Little Hans (1909*b*); it was also the fact that Hans loved his father and did not wish to lose him. His mother, moreover, though not realistically available as a sexual object, was not rejecting as a love object. Though a rival in terms of internal reality, his father was nevertheless a support and an object for identification as a real person. This conflict, in brief, is the first really significant confrontation to the child of the difference between external and internal reality. It is this difference which leads to mobilization of the signal anxiety which initiates the major defence of the future hysteric —repression.

It is my thesis that the true hysteric, whether male or female, has experienced a genuine triangular conflict. The hysteric, in addition, has been able to retain significant object relationships with both parents. Frequently, however, the post-oedipal relationship has been less satisfactory and more ambivalent than the relationship established in the pre-oedipal period. Hysterics, in brief, have paid too heavy a price for their attempted resolution of the oedipal triangle. They have nevertheless retained the potential capacity to recognize and tolerate internal reality and its wishes and conflicts, which they are capable of distinguishing from external reality. The patient's ability to distinguish these two aspects of reality is a major criterion for analysability and this may indeed constitute the essence of the capacity to distinguish between the therapeutic alliance and the transference neurosis.

It has, of course, long been recognized that the ability to modify primitive instinctual responses is initiated during the pre-oedipal years of development. The child first learns to tolerate delay and frustration in the early mother–child relationship. During the second, third and fourth years of life the child optimally acquires certain controls and achieves some degree of independence and autonomy. During this period, moreover, the child expands his capacity for one-to-one relationships, thus adding to his own ego identifications. The major developmental tasks during the pre-oedipal years include, first, the development of the capacity to accept certain limitations within one-to-one relationships without feeling rejected or devalued; second, toleration of increasing periods of separation from important objects (which involves taking added pleasure in available substitutes); and third, achievement of pleasure in active mastery and learning.

In all these tasks, the major frame of reference is the one-to-one relationship. The emergence of defences against primitive instinct is thus mainly initiated by the wish for approval and its negative counterpart—fear of disapproval. The major differences in the relation to the parents is in part attributable to their sexual differences. Their role in each of these three crucial areas is also highly significant. It is to be anticipated that the one to-one relationship with the mother will differ significantly from that with the father. Not only are their roles significantly different, but their spontaneous responses to the child's progression and regression will obviously cover an enormous range. It is almost inevitable that the child's relation with one of its parents will be more ambivalent than that with the other. Mastery of the hostility in the less good relationship will typically result in certain reaction formations. These, I would suggest, form the basis of the obsessional defences which all of us recognize as important concomitants of the character structure of the most analysable patients.

In this very brief outline it is impossible to attempt to describe the wide range of different problems confronting the little girl, as compared with the little boy. I will accordingly focus on the specific developmental hazards which appear to be determinants of the relatively high incidence of hysterical symptoms, whether true or so-called, in adult women. First, besides pathology in the mother, there are many reasons which increase the probability that the little girl's pre-oedipal relationship with her mother will be more ambivalent than that with her father. While in healthy development the little girl's identification with her mother will be the earliest one-to-one relationship, the oedipal conflict, however, specifically entails a shift of libidinal object choice for the little girl, and her first object, the mother, becomes her rival. It is easy to see how relative earlier failures will tend to impair the maintenance of a good object relationship between mother and daughter during the infantile neurosis, an impairment which may adversely affect the girl's feminine identification and the internalization of a positive ego-ideal.

It is also to be anticipated that many fathers are less demanding and more openly affectionate to their attractive little daughters than they are to their little sons. When this has been a striking feature of the pre-oedipal period, there may be an impairment of full genital development. The shift to the father is, moreover, immediately preceded by full recognition of sexual differences in the phase well described as both phallic and narcissistic. Earlier failures may thus compound penis envy, on the one hand; on the other, the girl may respond to her increased ambivalence by a regressive magnification of earlier passive needs.

The boy's identification with his father during the closing phases of the pre-oedipal period tends to reinforce his reaction formation against passivity. The analysable man who has failed adequately to resolve his oedipal situation is thus likely to present, at least initially, an obsessional rather than hysterical character structure or symptomatology. This same finding is, however, at least relatively true of the group I have described as the most analysable hysterical women. First, their positive identification with the mother's caretaking activity has often been apparent during the second and third years of life. Second, in my experience they have defensively reinforced penis envy and associated ambitions towards active achievement, partly in identification, but also in order to please a father who is not only an oedipal object but also the parent with whom the pre-oedipal relationship was less ambivalent and more stable.

Despite characteristic differences, men and women who have been successfully analysed share certain major developmental successes. The ability to achieve and maintain a positive therapeutic alliance and to work through the terminal phase has been seen to be optimal in patients whose analytic material has revealed substantial mastery of ambivalence in the early mother–child relationship. This usually entails the initiation and maintenance of certain reaction formations which prove to be prophylactic against significant ego regression during the establishment of the analytic situation. These patients had, in addition, consolidated genuine one-to-one relations with both of their parents before the onset of the genital oedipal situation. Their response to both the analytic situation and the transference neurosis has demonstrated a capacity to distinguish between external and internal reality. This capacity has been most crucially tested in respect of the regressive revival of a triangular oedipal conflict in the transference neurosis. They have demonstrated during the analytic process a sustained capacity to tolerate anxiety and depression. They have, finally, demonstrated the capacity to renounce without bitterness or self-devaluation the realistically unavailable and actively to approach and attempt to attain available objects and realistic ideals.

I will give here a vignette, not of any individual patient, but of the findings which would lead me to decide that a woman should be classified as a true hysteric who is ready for analysis. She is usually well past adolescence; she has usually completed her formal education, though she may be a graduate student. She is often a virgin; if not, she has been disappointed in her sexual experiences. Though she may have had brief periods of some promiscuity, she has usually given this up at the time she is seen. While she may not be frigid, she has not been able to make a major sexual investment in a man she cares for as a real person. Often she has somewhere in her life, and has sometimes already married, a man who is in love with her but to whom she cannot respond sexually. She often comes after something which might be described as an hour of truth. Some event or personal confrontation has at last made it clear to her that the problem lies within herself. One such patient, who was not quite ready when she first consulted me, attributed her difficulties to the absence of any appropriate men in the Boston area. It was only after she realized that this was a fallacy that she returned and commenced a supervised analysis. The opening stages of this patient's successful analysis are described in Chapter 11.

Most true hysterics and hysterical characters, though they have failed to achieve a mature heterosexual relationship, have been notably successful in the area of work. This is true of all the patients to whom I have given this diagnosis. All of these patients have, in addition, been able to make and keep friends. Many of them were the eldest, usually the most gifted, and typically the father's favourite child. None of them, as far as I can recall, have been only children. The father in most cases had idolized this daughter and boasted of her academic, personal and social successes. Although few of these patients described their fathers as actively seductive, they were usually aware of their fathers' investment in them.

In a number of these patients the failure to resolve a well-developed oedipal situation was at least partially attributable to external events. A father, for example, who had been very much in evidence during the child's first four or five years was lost, either permanently or for an extended period, at the height of the child's unresolved oedipal situation. One motive, namely maintenance and consolidation of the father–daughter relationship, was therefore absent at the critical period. Instead of mastery through neutralization, sublimation and positive identification with the mother, there occurred massive repression, with the oedipal father still unrelinquished and a major barrier to adult heterosexual object choice. Similarly, separation or loss of the mother during this critical period, by increasing the child's guilt, thereby impairs the achievement of a positive ego-ideal and identification.

How does this group of almost ideally analysable hysterics differ from the second category, the potential good hysterics? This second group includes a somewhat wider range of symptomatology and character structure than the first group. It is not therefore possible to give a specific clinical vignette. Generally speaking, however, they are usually younger, and are always less mature than the first group. They are often the youngest, and sometimes only children. They have failed to achieve ego-syntonic obsessional defences as stable as those seen in the first group. They are somewhat more passive and less consistent in their academic and professional achievements. Their friendships are less stable and more openly ambivalent. They are often afraid of their dependent wishes, which are nearer the surface than is typically the case with the true good hysteric.

The major problem in the analysis of this group of patients concerns the first phase of analysis; namely, the establishment of a stable analytic situation in which an analysable transference neurosis may gradually emerge. Some of them are quite simply too young to make a genuine commitment. Others, first seen in a state of neurotic decompensation, may respond to analysis in one of two ways; namely, flight into health, or the emergence of a regressive transference neurosis before the establishment of a therapeutic alliance. If, however, these pitfalls can be avoided, this group of patients prove able to achieve a genuine result. They do not necessarily present serious difficulties regarding either the emergence and analysis of the transference neurosis, or the working through of the terminal phase.

To give two very brief clinical examples:

A single, twenty-three-year-old graduate student applied for treatment because she was 'doing poorly at school and because of an unsatisfactory affair with a married man'. She had recently developed acute anxiety symptoms during an examination period and for the first time had done poorly in her academic work. This patient was the second of three children and the only girl. Her father was described as a passive, rather unsuccessful man, who occasionally seemed to be depressed. Her mother had a severe problem with drinking during the patient's adolescent years. The patient had dealt with this by becoming maternal and independent. She had always done well at school and had had a most successful college career at a well-known women's college. She had, however, always relied heavily on the approval of others. Her work habits had been somewhat erratic, and she had indulged in considerable destructive acting out in her heterosexual relations. On examination, she proved to be a friendly, warm young woman, whose desire for analysis was mainly motivated by her current decompensation and relatively severe anxiety.

This patient was accepted for supervised analysis. Fortunately she was referred to an extremely gifted woman therapist. The opening stages of her analysis proved to be stormy. Between her acceptance and the commencement of her analysis she had tried to stabilize her unsatisfactory life situation. She had great difficulty in tolerating anxiety without either acting out or attempting to control the analytic situation. For several months there was considerable doubt as to whether she would be able to develop a therapeutic alliance sufficiently secure to permit the working through of a transference neurosis. Eventually, however, her anxiety tolerance increased, she formed a stable therapeutic alliance and developed a highly analysable transference neurosis. The terminal stages of this patient's very successful analysis are described in Chapter 11.

A young woman aged twenty-one applied for analytic treatment because of her anxiety about heterosexual object relations. This patient was the youngest of three children. Her parents had been divorced during her early childhood. She had seen little of her father during her childhood and adolescence, but had recently seen him and developed very strong, somewhat sexualized fantasies after dancing with him. She did not describe any overt neurotic symptoms during childhood and adolescence. She had however, been a somewhat dependent child, who had experienced anxiety about leaving home on a number of occasions. Her school record was adequate but in no way outstanding. She was not very ambitious except for marriage and motherhood. Up to the time of referral, however, there had been few serious heterosexual relationships.

This patient was referred for a supervised analysis with some hesitation. It was felt that she was very immature and possibly not yet prepared to make a serious commitment. Although she expressed superficial co-operation during her initial interview, it soon proved that these fears had been correct. The patient raised innumerable problems about the arrangements for her analysis. She questioned whether she needed such intensive treatment. Within less than a month after her referral the analysis was interrupted by mutual agreement.

The last two of my four groups comprise the vast majority of so-called 'good' hysterics. In one of them, depressive characters are typically women who have signally failed to mobilize their active resources during every important developmental crisis. Some of them may be analysable in a long and difficult analysis. Their basic self-esteem is low, and in addition they tend to devalue their own femininity. Despite these serious drawbacks, many of these patients have experienced some genuine triangular conflict, often idealizing their fathers to an excessive degree. They have usually failed to develop adequate reaction formations during the pre-oedipal period. While, in briefest terms, they are able to recognize and tolerate considerable depression, they have failed significantly in the area of mastery. They are not only passive; they also feel helpless. Despite these handicaps, they are often attractive, gifted women, whose depression is hidden by laughter and flirtation. Their manifest symptoms may be obviously hysterical.

It may be extremely difficult to recognize depressive characters at the time of initial evaluation. Often, however, they first come to the attention of the psychiatrist or analyst at a somewhat later age than those included in my other groups. The fact that they did not seek help earlier is seldom as attributable to lack of opportunity as it is to their lack of basic self-esteem. They are often first seen when they are practically defeated, with considerable impairment of major ego functions. These patients typically verbalize feelings of helplessness and depression quite early in treatment. They tend to develop passive, dependent transference reactions which impair their capacity adequately to distinguish between therapeutic alliance and the transference neurosis. Such patients should not be referred for traditional analysis without careful assessment, which should include their total life situation and its potential for progressive alteration. All of these patients, in my own clinical experience, present serious problems during the terminal phases of analysis. Unless, therefore, there are positive, available realistic goals, they may drift into a relatively interminable analytic situation.

To give one brief example: A married woman of thirty-six was referred for analysis with the presenting symptoms of frigidity, social insecurity and occasional depression. She had been married for ten years to a difficult, somewhat withdrawn husband. She had two children, who appeared to be relatively well adjusted. This patient was the youngest of four children by some five years. She was the third girl and had always felt that her birth had been an accident, doubly compounded by her parents' desire for another boy. In addition, her parents were Jews who wished to be accepted in the non-Jewish community. All her siblings were relatively fair, with non-Semitic features. Her next eldest sister was an attractive blue-eyed blonde. The patient, however, was markedly Semitic in appearance, with a large nose and dark, curly hair. The patient stated that she had felt rejected by her mother and next eldest sister for as long as she could remember. She had, however, been loved and accepted by her father, who was less involved in the break from Judaism. Her father, however, had died suddenly just before the patient's eighth birthday. Her mother subsequently went to work to support the family. The patient herself was sent to boarding school before she was ten years old. She remembers her vacations at home as periods of loneliness and exclusion from the activities of the rest of the family. At school, however, she had been active and successful, obtaining a far higher education than any of her siblings. She had achieved considerable success in her professional career before her marriage.

This marriage clearly revealed her own identification with her family's rejection of Judaism. Her husband was non-Jewish, and fair and blonde like her elder sister. The marriage, however, had not been very satisfactory. She had never been able to obtain sexual gratification. She was unable to feel socially secure because of her Semitic appearance. She was subject to occasional periods of depression and lethargy, which reminded her acutely of the vacation periods during her childhood and adolescence.

This patient developed an extremely intense transference neurosis before she had established a genuine therapeutic alliance. Her transference was marked by extreme dependence, sense of rejection and outbursts of anxiety. Over the course of a very extended analysis this patient showed considerable improvement in several areas. She made immeasurable gains in respect of her social insecurity. She returned to her professional career and obtained considerable gratification from her outstanding success. Her sexual symptoms showed relatively little change. She remained subject to periods of depression, which were particularly evident during every analytic vacation. Although this patient was able to utilize her analysis for many positive gains, she proved genuinely unable fully to work through a successful termination. It proved necessary to see her from time to time for many years after the completion of her analytic treatment. Like the patient described in Chapter 6, she realized that her depressive episodes could be considerably modified if she arranged occasional interviews with her former analyst. It must be emphasized that this highly gifted woman continued throughout the analysis and after it to function at an extremely high level outside of the analytic situation. She remained nevertheless a vulnerable, depressive character, whose continued adaptation was contingent on the availability of some realistic support.

Fourth and last is the group of so-called 'good' hysterics, typically characterized by a symptomatic picture which can only be described as floridly hysterical. This group of patients overlaps considerably with Easser and Lesser's 'hysteroids'. However, while their symptoms may present a façade which looks genital they prove in treatment to be incapable of recognizing or tolerating a genuine triangular situation. For them, as for Oedipus himself, the parent of the same sex has not remained a real object in any meaningful way. Such patients all too readily express intense sexualized transference fantasies. They tend, however, to regard such fantasies as potential areas of realistic gratification. They are genuinely incapable of the meaningful distinction between external and internal reality which is prequisite to the establishment of a therapeutic alliance and the emergence of an analysable transference neurosis.

To give one very brief clinical example of the type of transference which characterizes many so-called good hysterics:

One of the first patients whose analysis I supervised in Boston came with a presenting symptom of frigidity. There was clear evidence of an intense, unresolved oedipal attachment to her father, which was amply confirmed during the first months of an analysis conducted as a candidate's first control case. The patient developed an intense sexualized transference but showed relatively little evidence of a genuine therapeutic alliance. In addition, there was considerable evidence that her capacity for genuine object relations was shallow and narcissistic. The analysis nevertheless appeared to progress uneventfully for some months. Then one day the patient entered the analyst's office and said: 'Before I lie down, I would like to get one thing straight. If I divorce my husband will you divorce your wife and marry me?'

In this somewhat devastating confrontation the patient clearly revealed her inability to distinguish between transference and reality. She was genuinely incapable of recognizing, let alone accepting, the fact that the analyst was realistically unavailable. She had never relinquished the hope for her father, had in fact left all her most treasured possessions in the parental home at the time she married. While this patient's presenting symptoms were classically hysterical, her attachment to her father was of a nature which excluded her mother as a meaningful object. She had not, in brief, achieved the pre-oedipal relations with both parents which are an essential prerequisite for true as compared to so-called hysteria.

So-called good hysterics do not, in my opinion, meet the criteria for traditional psychoanalysis. Their major pathology is attributable to significant developmental failure in basic ego functions. Initially they may, however, sometimes prove difficult to distinguish from more analysable women who have regressed during the period which preceded their referral. Extended evaluation will often prove invaluable in making the distinction. The more analysable patients often reconstitute fairly rapidly. The so-called good hysteric will tend, conversely, rapidly to develop an intense sexualized transference even in a structured face-to-face interview situation.

These women may first be seen at almost any age. Frequently they have been seen by more than one previous therapist or analyst, with unfavourable results. Unlike patients in the other groups, they have few available areas of past or present conflict-free interest or autonomous ego functions. They seldom present a history which includes a genuine period of latency in respect of either achievement or peer relationships. Their obsessional defences, if present, are not directed against their own ego-alien impulses. Like the obsessional defences of borderline or psychotic patients, they are directed towards ensuring their perception and control of certain aspects of external reality.

In many cases the developmental history will reveal one or more of the following findings:

(1) absence of, or significant separation from, one or both parents during the first four years of life;

(2) serious pathology in one or both parents, often associated with an unhappy or broken marriage;

(3) serious and/or prolonged physical illness in childhood;

(4) a continuing hostile dependent relationship with the mother, who is either devalued or seen as rejecting and devaluing;

(5) absence of meaningful, sustained object relations with either sex.

None of these observations is sufficient by itself to reach the diagnosis of so-called good hysteria. Two or more of them combined with a regressive transference readiness should, however, constitute a warning signal.

The basic question I have posed in this chapter may be stated quite simply: How far can we regard manifest oedipal or genital symptomatology (i.e. instinctual content) as acceptable evidence that the patient in question has achieved or maintained a level of ego development at which the capacity for identification, object relations and affect tolerance permits emergence and recognition of a triangular situation which involves three whole individuals? This I regard as indispensable in determining potential ability to distinguish between external and internal reality, which is one major criterion of analysability.

I have attempted in this chapter to indicate certain subgroups which may be distinguished among female patients whose presenting symptoms are hysterical. All of these patients initially presented a clinical picture clearly suggestive of an unresolved oedipal genital situation. Not all of them proved to be analysable hysterics. I may, in conclusion, paraphrase my opening jingle:

> There are many little girls
> Whose complaints are little pearls
> Of the classical hysterical neurotic.
> And when this is true
> Analysis can and should ensue,
> But when this is false
> 'Twill be chaotic.

15

A DEVELOPMENTAL MODEL AND THE THEORY OF THERAPY[1]

(1965)

The essential core of clinical psychoanalysis is the revival of early conflicts through the medium of the transference neurosis. For this to occur, backward movement involving both wishes and memories is an essential prerequisite. Regression, in brief, must precede the new and better resolution of intrapsychic conflict which represents a primary therapeutic goal. The inevitability of such regression has frequently been discussed in psychoanalytic literature. In Chapter 10, for example, differing opinions as to its significance, value and technical handling were discussed in some detail. The need to revive and work through conflicts characteristic of early stages of development was considered essential by many authors. It is nevertheless widely agreed that certain forms of regression may represent major determinants of interminable or unsuccessful analysis. In view of this problem, the differentiation between different types and degrees of regression in the special one-to-one relationship integral to the analytic situation may be approached within the context of psychoanalysis as a general developmental psychology.

There have been few who have contributed more to this aspect of psychoanalysis than Heinz Hartmann. His monograph *Ego Psychology and the Problem of Adaptation*, though it did not become available in English until 1958, has widely influenced psychoanalytic ego psychology since 1939. His later contributions (cf. 1951, 1952, 1954) have expanded and enriched the concept of the adaptive hypothesis which is now included by most theorists as one of our basic metapsychological assumptions. In addition,

[1] Presented in draft form in the panel 'The Theory of the Therapeutic Process' at the Fall meeting of the American Psychoanalytic Association in December 1963. The model used in the paper was also presented in the Symposium on 'Classification' at the 22nd Congress of the International Psycho-Analytical Association, Edinburgh, in 1961. First published in the *Int. J. Psycho-Anal.* (1965), **46**.

these papers reveal Hartmann's consistent efforts to include in his discussion findings relevant to psychic development acquired by other individuals and by methods based on other frames of reference.

In Chapter 7 I discussed the nature and function of unconscious mental content and its relation to mental processes comprised within Hartmann's definition of the 'conflict-free sphere of the ego' (1939). That chapter focused primarily on a comparison between the contributions of Hartmann, Kris, Loewenstein and Rapaport on the one hand, and those of Melanie Klein and her school on the other. More general questions, however, were raised as to the impact of the growing body of knowledge relevant to the role of early object relations on our conceptual assumptions. I therefore suggested that it may become necessary to modify our conceptual framework to take fully into account the object needs of the human infant and that 'it may indeed prove that psychoanalytic truth cannot be adequately expressed in abstract conceptual terms based on the individual psychic apparatus'. I concluded, however, that 'we have by no means exhausted the possibilities of conceptual reformulation and [that] the role of object relations in early infancy still remains open to debate'.

In his paper 'Technical Implications of Ego Psychology' Hartmann suggested: 'if we let our curiosity tempt us to look into the future, we may say that technical progress might depend on a more systematic study of the various functional units within the ego' (1951). Here as elsewhere Hartmann indicates the close relationship in his own mind between empirical clinical material and basic developmental hypotheses. In this chapter I should like to explore somewhat further the possibilities for conceptual reformulation, attempting to include within our theory of individual development certain specific hypotheses relevant to the role of early object relations in initiating definitive aspects of ego structure and function. Consideration of the significance of regression in the analytic situation may in this context represent an effort to consider 'the various functional units within the ego' from a developmental point of view.

In a recent discussion I said:

Our developmental hypothesis includes by definition both progressive and regressive potentialities at all times. This statement applies both to instinctual development and to the structured ego–superego system. . . . It is not by chance that Freud postulated the infantile neurosis as a general developmental phenomenon. . . . Symptoms may in this context represent a necessary step backwards preceding conflict solution and progressive character formation. Consolidation, in contrast, of primitive or regressive defences into the post-oedipal character structure represents an important genetic factor in neurotic character formation (Zetzel, 1964, pp. 153–4).

As this statement implies, the regressive features integral to the analytic situation, like the regressive features which characterize all maturational changes, may be defined as potentially adaptive. However, just as psychic development presents regressive hazards, so, too, the regressive components integral to the transference neurosis present well-recognized dangers. The theory of the psychoanalytic process, it is suggested, may thus be considered in relation to our theory of the developmental process itself. It is a major premise, in this context, that a crucial differentiation be made between those ego attributes which determine the capacity for sustained motivation towards progressive maturational achievement, and those ego defences which must be substantially renounced during the course of transference analysis.

The major assumptions underlying this discussion of the theory of therapy may be summarized as follows: Early experience and the quality and stability of the object relations achieved play a central role in initiating early ego identifications. Such identifications play a significant role in determining the setting in which the individual reaches a level of maturation at which he is potentially capable of tolerating frustration, delay and separation. Between this earliest period and the onset of the oedipal situation occurs the period of individual psychological development which determines the capacity to enter and genuinely experience the oedipal situation itself; which, second, influences the nature of the resolution attempted or achieved; and, as a result, the predisposition to different types of regression in adult life. Finally, and most important for this discussion, it probably determines the potential capacity to develop, work through and resolve an analysable transference neurosis.

In his paper 'Problems of Infantile Neurosis' (1954) Heinz

Hartmann mentioned the many factors which influence 'the form and intensity of object relationships in the development of the ego'. He suggested, however, that there are 'missing links between these very early happenings and what we know now about the aetiological significance of later phases'. He is here referring to much the same area which I discussed in 'Symptom Formation and Character Formation':

> our theory has not as yet clearly conceptualized the meeting-point and the overlap between pregenital experience and the infantile neurosis. . . . There is wide recognition, first, of the importance of early experience, and second, of the relatively late acquisition of signal anxiety as the motive of defence. The many crucial developmental aspects, however, of the period intervening between self-object differentiation and the classical infantile neurosis remain open to questions and differences of opinion (Zetzel, 1964, p. 151; see also Chapter 16).

It should go without saying, but unfortunately does not always do so, that both the theory and the technique of clinical psychoanalysis are based on the concept of intrapsychic conflict which has been fundamental to our discipline from the time that Freud first postulated a dynamic process of repression and the dynamic, instinctual nature of what is repressed. In particular, the significance of repression and related defences in closing off and rendering inaccessible fantasies, wishes and associated memories, direct emergence of which would produce an internal danger situation, suggests an area of individual mental life contained within a relatively closed system. It is now recognized that signal anxiety as the motive for repression and related defences can only develop when psychic structure and function have reached a level at which internal signals of danger can be recognized. In clinical psychoanalysis, therefore, major manifestations of the transference neurosis and the analytic process involve the recognition, tolerance and mastery of the manifest anxiety mobilized by the fantasies and impulses which present specific internal dangers. This can only occur if previously stable neurotic defences are gradually undermined, i.e. become less successful in maintaining a relatively closed system.

To accomplish this the analytic process requires of the patient a capacity to regress to a degree sufficient to permit the reopening of conflicts previously closed off by those defences which represent unconscious automatic responses to signal anxiety. Such regression mainly involves a gradual diminution of automatic unconscious ego defences. This entails significant re-emergence of early intrapsychic conflict. It need not, however, necessarily impinge on reality testing or result in the re-emergence of more primitive mental processes which diminish the capacity for sustained object relations. In other words, a distinction must be made between regression involving the defensive ego and related instinctual content, and regression which undermines basic ego capacities. Successful psychoanalysis requires, first, the capacity to relinquish neurotic ego defences in the service of future maturation, and second, sufficient mastery of the developmental processes which concern early object relations and early ego development to minimize the possibility of serious ego regression. The capacity, in brief, to differentiate fantasy and transference from reality must be maintained. Regression affecting ego capacities in this latter area may obliterate the capacity to separate therapeutic alliance from the transference neurosis. This capacity is to be regarded as an indispensable feature of the analytic process.

In a number of papers Heinz Hartmann has discussed from many different points of view his concept of secondary autonomy of the ego. Primary autonomy, it might be suggested, concerns those ego capacities which, in the absence of serious pathology, will develop spontaneously without necessarily involving internal mastery of conflict. Certain innate attributes play a considerable part in determining individual differences in such capacities as tolerance of delay, anxiety and frustration. Secondary autonomy, like secondary anxiety, secondary identification and/or secondary narcissism, implies more individualized contributions determining qualitative differences. Although Hartmann suggests that definitive ego characteristics which possess secondary autonomy are more stable than ego defences, he nevertheless makes it abundantly clear that these qualities may be subject to regression under certain circumstances. Such regression, he also indicates, will include related modification in the instinctual energy available for autonomous ego functions. Neutralized energy, in short, will be re-sexualized or re-aggressified as secondary autonomy is regressively impaired.

Hartmann's paper 'The Mutual Influences in the Development of Ego and Id' (1952) clearly recognizes the complex relationship between structure and function implicit in the concept of secondary autonomy. He not only suggests the need to differentiate among types and degrees of neutralization, but also relates the degree of secondary autonomy to 'the resistivity of ego functions against regression'. 'Various functions of the ego', he says, 'may achieve various degrees of virtual independence from conflicts and from regressive tendencies in various individuals.' He notes, moreover, the relevance of consistent object relations to these crucial questions, saying, 'The development of consistent object relations on the one hand facilitates, but on the other also depends on neutralization.' It may thus be suggested that a developmental approach to the theory of therapy must inevitably take into consideration the continuing significance of the capacity for constant object relations. Successful analysis, it would generally be agreed, results in an increased capacity for all that is implied in the concept of neutralization. It has also become increasingly evident that one of the most important prerequisites concerns the pre-existence of a degree of secondary autonomy which will substantially militate against the regression of basic ego functions. A comprehensive theory of the therapeutic process must therefore take into consideration all those factors which contribute to secondary autonomy on the one hand, and on the other, the concomitant facilitation of partial regression which is integral to the development and resolution of the transference neurosis.

As my title suggests, I hope to illustrate certain aspects of the therapeutic process by means of a developmental model of the psychic apparatus. Since this discussion is mainly confined to clinical psychoanalysis, I will focus on the analysis of patients whose earliest development has been sufficiently successful to make them potentially capable of developing and resolving an analysable transference neurosis. It will be necessary at the same time to indicate, for contrast and comparison, the developmental abnormalities which may present significant barriers to both the development of the analytic situation (therapeutic alliance) and the emergence and resolution of a genuine transference neurosis.

Figure 1 illustrates those stages of earliest development which,

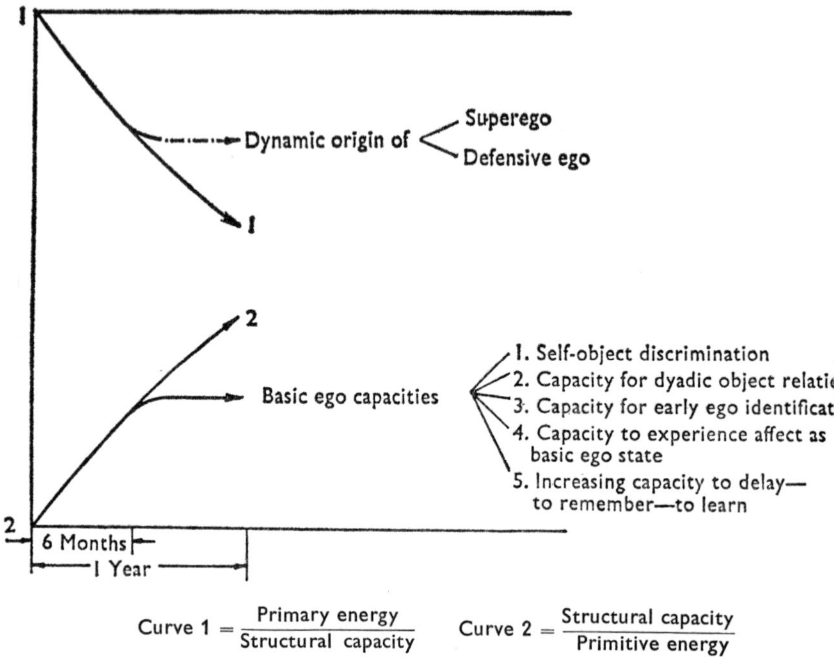

FIG. 1

it is proposed, substantially determine the basic psychic equipment with which the individual child enters the decisive period of infantile development which intervenes between the achievement of self-object differentiation and the resolution of the infantile neuroses. The base-line refers to time. The vertical axis is more complex. Starting from left to right, the upper curve represents the relation of unstructured energy to which the psychic apparatus is exposed with available structural capacities to control, modify, dismiss or gratify the stimuli which impinge from internal and external sources. The lower curve, which is a reciprocal to the upper one, represents the relation of structural capacities to unstructured energy. For purposes of this discussion it is assumed that structural capacities are negligible at birth. This is in keeping with Freud's definition of primary anxiety. The infant reacts with immediate, uncontrolled responses to all stimuli which disturb his equilibrium. During the early months of life, both maturation and perceptual experience lead to a gradual relative increase in structural capacities, the precursors of that part of the definitive ego to which Heinz Hartmann has assigned primary autonomy. These include the ability to direct instinctual activity towards specific sources of gratification, to tolerate delay, and increasingly, the capacity to internalize (i.e. to remember and integrate past experiences, both of a pleasurable and of a painful nature).

This illustration proceeds up to the time of life, subject to individual variations, at which the infant has become capable of self-object differentiation and a stable object relationship with one person, usually the mother. Such recognition implicitly includes some integration of the gratifying feeding mother and her rejecting and/or punitive counterpart. It is a major premise of this discussion that certain characteristics of definitive psychic structure are significantly influenced by the nature and quality of the early stages of ego development which culminate during the period of self-object differentiation. By necessity, the infant will have been exposed to both positive and negative experiences (i.e. gratification and frustration). It is proposed that stable, satisfactory self-object differentiation is contingent on earlier experience, however determined (i.e. innate or experiential), which has been on the whole qualitatively positive. This by no means implies absence of negative experience; it does, however, imply that positive should optimally outweigh negative during the early months of life. I suggest that this facilitates a positive object relationships and that these form the nucleus around which develop ego functions possessing secondary autonomy.

Now the qualities most relevant to the analytic situation concern:

(i) The capacity to maintain basic trust in the absence of immediate gratification.

(ii) The capacity to maintain self-object differentiation in the absence of a loved object.

(iii) The potential capacity to accept realistic limitations. This concerns both personal lack of omnipotence and, conversely, recognition that failure on the part of the object to meet wishes and demands may not derive from hostility or rejection but from realistic limitations which must be accepted.

That aspect of basic psychic equipment, therefore, which throughout life will form the core around which major ego functions develop, particularly those comprised under the definition 'secondary autonomy', is here illustrated as the lower of the two reciprocal curves. The significance of its reciprocal (namely, the upper curve) is of course of at least equal importance. The point marked '1' on this illustration concerns in essence the nature and quantity of unaltered primitive instinct which will remain minimally available for either neutralization, sublimation or direct external discharge. Such energy is destined for later incorporation in the definitive superego and/or unconscious ego defences of the individual. The well-recognized pregenital precursors of the superego are thus here illustrated, with particular reference to both the quality and quantity of unmodified instinctual energy involved. Here, too, the relative preponderance of positive or negative experience must be taken into consideration. Individual differences in both innate endowment (with respect to instinctual endowment and to the area of autonomous ego functions) and in actual perceptual experience may substantially influence the quality of the infant's subjective experience. Whatever the reason, however, it may be stated with some conviction that the greater the positive experience the higher the level at which point '2', i.e. self-object differentiation, is achieved—and, conversely, the lower point '1', i.e. the amount of unaltered instinctual energy with which the individual will be endowed.

Figure 2 continues the developmental process as it might be visualized in optimal maturation. The line parallel to the baseline shown in the lower half of the model represents the core around which the autonomous ego develops. Its parallel in the upper half indicates both the early source and the continued significance of the primitive instinctual energy which contributes to the superego and/or unconscious ego defences. These two parallel lines thus comprise that part of basic psychic equipment which is least subject to significant modification during later maturational phases. Progressive changes concern the acquisition of additional ego-syntonic energy at later levels of development. Substantial regression in the lower of these two lines implies progressively diminished self-esteem, impaired capacity for object relations, and ultimately, loss of self-object differentiation. Such regression may readily be compared to Hartmann's many references to regressively impaired secondary autonomy

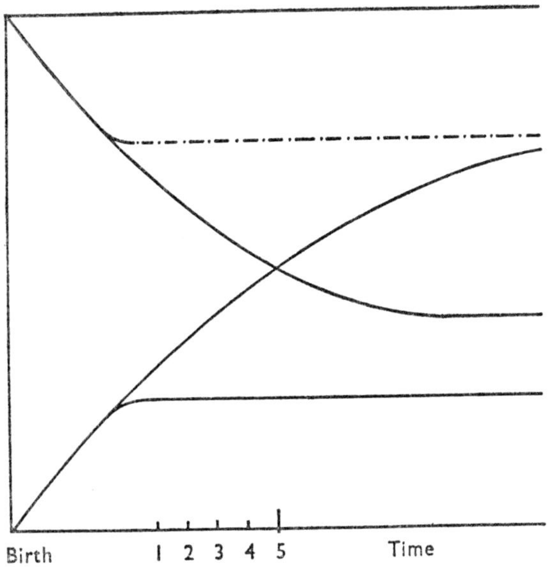

Curves 1 and 2 cross approximately age 5 (resolution of oedipal situation)

FIG. 2

of the ego. Concurrent regression in the upper line will mean an increase in the unmodified instinctual energy available to the superego, which increase characterizes most depressive states. The line will later show the regressive impairment of superego functions which accompanies significant loss of self-object differentiation in overt psychosis.

Proceeding along the two reciprocal curves to the point at which they meet, this portion of the developmental model includes the period of time which intervenes between the achievement of self-object differentiation and the time at which the psychic apparatus has become capable not only of initiating but also of maintaining stable intrapsychic defences involving signal anxiety. In optimal development, it may be suggested that the passing of the oedipal situation substantially coincides with the time at which the psychic apparatus is stimulated towards this goal to a substantial degree.

During this period there is a gradual increase in structural attributes relative to unmodified primitive instinct. Although for purposes of clarity the curves are shown as smoothly progressive, there are a number of complex factors which require some amplification. For example, during approximately the first three years of life object relations are predominantly dyadic. Although the healthy child is able to achieve good object relations with more than one person, rivalry situations remain essentially pre-oedipal, i.e. for gratification and/or mastery in respect of one person at a time. Moreover, a major problem in the modification of primitive instinct during this time involves the mastery of aggression and its concomitants. Optimal development of autonomous ego functions thus concerns, first, further integration and security of basic identifications; second, increased motivation towards learning and mastery; and, third, further renunciation of demands for total gratification.

The onset of the oedipal situation is here only indicated by the passage of time. It is, however, also marked by qualitative changes in the nature and amount of unmodified instinctual energy and by a more complex (triadic) capacity for object relations. On the one hand, the genital period is marked by a definitive increase of unmodified sexual energies. This, however, is counterbalanced in the potentially healthy child by the positive one-to-one relations already established in relation to both parents. The emergence and resolution of the oedipal situation involve, first, the capacity to initiate and maintain stable intrapsychic defences in the face of ego-alien instinctual wishes predominantly oedipal in content; second, concurrent integration, within the sphere of both autonomous ego and ego-ideal, of a positive identification with the parent of the same sex; third, the renunciation of sexualized goals in respect of the parent of the opposite sex, yet at the same time strengthening an aim-inhibited positive object relationship; fourth, neutralization, sublimation or displacement of the aggression mobilized by rivalry with the parent of the same sex. Anxiety, i.e. fear, is one significant motive towards the initiation of defensive ego functions. It must also, however, be emphasized that it is not only fear and hate, but also love and trust which lead to all that is involved in mature resolution of this crucial conflict.

In healthy development, it is suggested, the crossing of the two reciprocal curves coincides with resolution of the oedipal conflict. At this time the primitive instinctual energy represented by the upper parallel line becomes consistently available to the unconscious defensive ego–superego system. In this illustration, however, it should be noted that the superego line is not very far above that of the defensive ego. Relatively little unmodified instinctual energy is available to the definitive superego of healthy individuals.

The crossing of the two reciprocal curves marks the following well-known psychoanalytic propositions:

(i) The close relationship between stable defences stimulated by signal anxiety and the resolution of the oedipal situation.

(ii) The classical definition of the definitive superego as the heir to the oedipal situation (i.e. the punitive aspect of the perceived parent of the same sex is incorporated in the unconscious superego).

(iii) The amnesia relevant to the events of the infantile neurosis which, following the cross-over, are typically relegated to the area of mental life which Freud originally defined as the repressed unconscious.

To the right of the cross-over, the area between the two reciprocal curves comprises wishes, fantasies and memories contained within a relatively closed system. The area between the lower curve and the ego base-line includes those ego functions to which Hartmann ascribes both primary and secondary autonomy. The instinctual energy available to this part of the ego, whatever its degree of consciousness, operates in an essentially open system. Included here are neutralized instinctual energy, both sexual and aggressive; instinctual energy modified by displacement or sublimation; and finally, primitive instinctual energy which has remained essentially ego-syntonic. Healthy development, in brief, requires not only the capacity to form stable ego defences, but also the successful modification and utilization of instinctual energies for adaptive purposes. It may also be suggested that secondary autonomy as here defined includes the capacity to recognize and tolerate affect, particularly anxiety and depression, and the related ability to permit some regression, i.e. partial reopening of the relatively closed system, without substantial concomitant impairment of the autonomous ego. Such regression, as is well known, not only includes neurotic symptom formation, dreams and fantasies, but also regression in the service of the ego, as defined by Ernst Kris (1950).

It should also be noted that the regressive components of major maturational changes, among which psychoanalysis may be included, may be differentiated as to which part of this model is affected. Instinctual regression resulting from increase of unmodified instinctual energy within the relatively closed system will lead to simultaneous movement of both reciprocal curves to the left. Such movement involves, first, the mobilization of anxiety, and second, a partial reopening in so far as the instinctual energy in question exceeds the specific defensive capacity of the ego to contain it. Such regression is nevertheless consistent with the maintenance of considerable secondary autonomy, provided that the lower base-line does not drop significantly. But if this occurs, regression has not only undermined ego defences but has also impaired basic ego functions. While instinctual regression may thus be regarded as potentially adaptive, ego regression usually implies more ominous changes.

This model, which illustrates optimal development, is of course hypothetical. It may nevertheless also serve to illustrate the major goals of therapeutic psychoanalysis, which may be regarded as a partial but adaptively modified revival and repetition of major aspects of the original developmental process. Before discussing the theory of therapy in more detail I will briefly indicate some possible variations in the mode of development which may lead to pathological symptomatology or character structure in adult life.

The next illustration (Figure 3), for example, concerns the developmental variations which may lead to a classical transference neurosis with hysterical symptomatology. In this model the development of basic psychic equipment has been on the whole satisfactory. The position of the two parallel lines, in other words, does not differ significantly from that shown in hypothetically healthy development. The variation concerns the rate of convergence and crossing of the two reciprocal curves. Predisposition to hysteria involves the establishment of powerful intrapsychic defences during the height of the oedipal conflict. This is illustrated by the earlier cross-over of the two reciprocal curves. Such premature closure implies that at least one of the goals involved in optimal resolution of the oedipal situation has not been achieved. Oedipal fantasies, in brief, have thus been subjected to repression and its related defences more than they

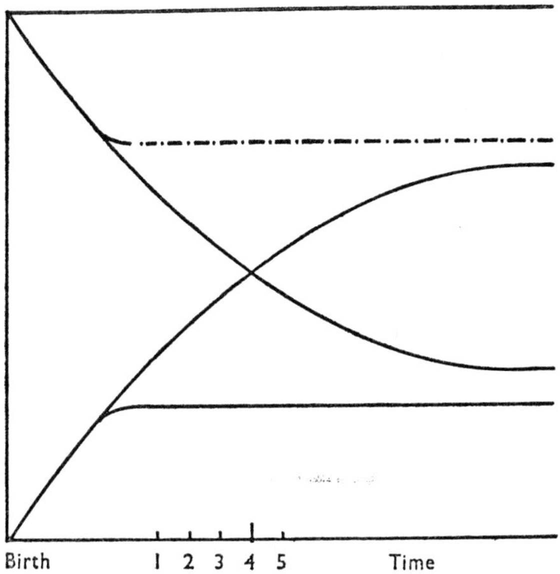

Curves 1 and 2 cross approximately age 4 (premature resolution of oedipal situation)

FIG. 3

have been mastered, modified or genuinely renounced. As a result, the area contained within the relatively closed system is proportionately greater. This inevitably implies that a smaller area is assigned to the open system which has been related to secondary autonomy. Less energy, both neutralized and unneutralized, is thus available to the autonomous ego. This may also imply a less stable integration of positive ego identification with the parent of the same sex.

In the future obsessional neurotic who is susceptible to transference neurosis, the hypothetical model would be very similar. The convergence and crossing of the two reciprocal curves, however, would be even more premature, occurring during the one-to-one relationships which characterize the first three years of life. Such premature crossing again implies an over-large area within the relatively closed system. The time of closure, in addition, also indicates the initiation and maintenance of major ego defences against aggression at its height—during the anal sadistic period. While some of the defences in question are consistent with and necessary for healthy development, they do not achieve a dominant position in the definitive psychic structure of healthy individuals. The models are by no means to be regarded as mutually exclusive but rather as illustrative of dominant trends.

The psychopathology of symptom neurosis thus concerns primarily the period of psychic development which follows self-object differentiation. Such psychopathology, however, may occur in individuals whose mastery of earlier developmental tasks is subject to wide variation. In individuals for whom psychoanalysis is definitely the treatment of choice, basic equipment is in general within normal limits. Secondary autonomy, though it may be restricted as a result of precocious development similar to that shown in obsessional conditions, is relatively stable and not therefore readily subject to regressive impairment. The goal of therapeutic psychoanalysis in such cases is primarily directed towards modification of the position of the two reciprocal curves. As a result of successful analysis, in brief, Figure 3 might represent the state of affairs at the beginning of treatment. The analytic process, in so far as it involves innumerable partial re-openings of the relatively closed area, facilitates more adaptive resolution of intrapsychic conflict. On completion of analysis, therefore, the model illustrating healthy development should be approximated.

It must be remembered, however, that even individuals whose basic equipment is essentially sound remain subject to regressive impairment of secondary autonomy under specific stress situations. Such regression in the analytic situation should be differentiated from the instinctual regression which is a concomitant of transference analysis. The significance of basic psychic equipment for the analytic situation is indicated in the next illustrations which concern more serious deviations from the hypothetical norm.

Figure 4 illustrates, perhaps in a somewhat exaggerated form, a developmental pattern which may be consistent with so-called normality for long periods of time. Precocious development of ego defences is indicated by a rate of convergence which results in very premature cross-over. Major defences are thus likely to compress reaction formation, intellectualization and isolation. Such development, however, is here associated with a basic psychic equipment which is not within normal limits. Self-object

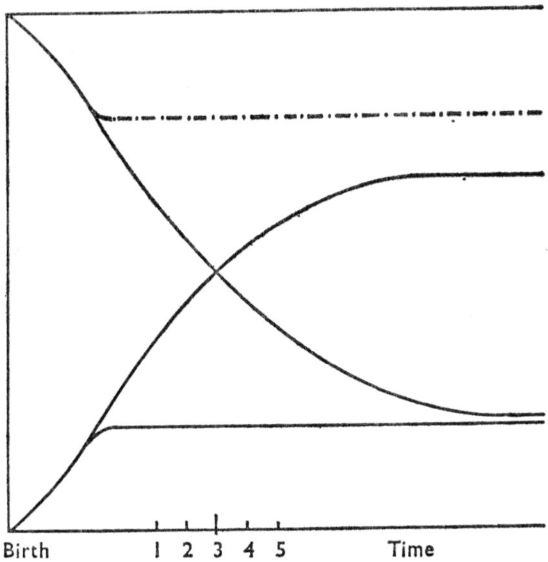

Precocious early development A. Low base-line (poor ego identification) B. High upper horizontal (archaic superego) C. Premature crossing of curves 1 and 2

FIG. 4

differentiation has taken place in a setting which limited the integration of a positive ego identification. Basic trust is not secure and is therefore vulnerable to narcissistic injury. The reciprocal height of the upper horizontal line indicates the greater quantity of unmodified instinctual energy within the superego–defensive ego system. It may also be noted that the greater distance between the superego and defensive ego area is consistent with the harsh, demanding superego typical of certain obsessional characters.

The relative steepness of the two reciprocal curves is in keeping with the rapid regression which may occur during decompensation of obsessional characters. The vulnerability of the autonomous ego and the related severity of the superego illustrate the predisposition to depressive illness long associated with obsessional character structure. Secondary autonomy in such individuals is not only restricted in many areas; it is also more readily vulnerable to regressive change as ego defences become precarious. The associated failure in basic trust has not only affected the original developmental process, but also presents serious problems in the establishment of a therapeutic alliance. Lack of secure positive ego identification, precocious initiation of stable ego defences, and a demanding superego foster intolerance of passivity and a related premium on mastery and achievement. Individuals whose developmental pattern approaches this illustration thus often present a deceptive façade of normality and health.

The last drawing (Figure 5) illustrates a possible development predisposing to more serious types of regression. In this figure, as in the preceding figure, basic psychic equipment has not resulted in stable self-object differentiation or a secure positive object relationship. The identification associated with the initiation of secondary autonomy of the ego is in both significantly vulnerable to narcissistic injury and regressive impairment. The obsessional character, however, has been stimulated towards precocious ego development, leading to premature closure and a relatively preponderant closed system. This is in keeping with the strong ego defences many such patients present against regression in the service of the ego. In contrast, the development of structure depicted in Figure 5 has been so inadequate during the later stages of infantile development that the capacity to respond to signal anxiety within a relatively closed system is almost non-existent. Unneutralized instinctual energy closely impinges at all times on an ego which has achieved a minimal degree of secondary autonomy. This indicates a vulnerability to regress to a level at which the capacity to differentiate between fantasy and reality can barely be maintained.

Both of these illustrations concern developmental failure which may, in some patients, contraindicate psychoanalysis as the treatment of choice. In the obsessional character with poor basic psychic equipment it may prove almost impossible to achieve a sufficiently secure therapeutic alliance to facilitate the undoing of ego defences established and maintained with excessive investment. Such patients, though they may go through the forms of analytic work, may be too heavily defended to permit the emergence of an analysable transference neurosis. In the borderline or potential psychotic case illustrated in Figure 5, in contrast, the relative failure of closure may be consistent with presenting symptomatology of manifest oedipal content and a

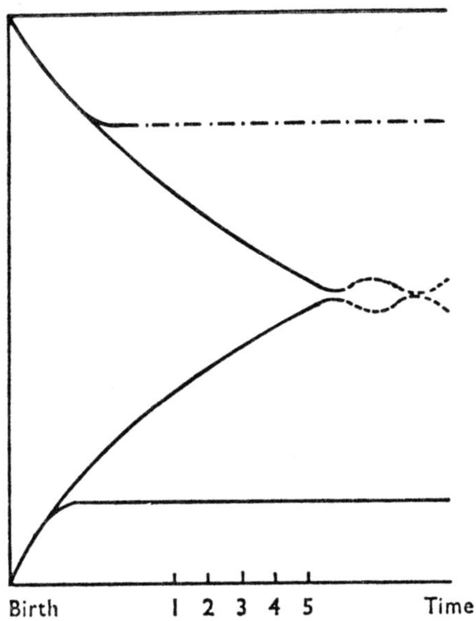

Relative development failure A. Low base-line. Insecure self-object differentiation B. Self-esteem low C. No stable crossing of curves 1 and 2

Fig. 5

deceptive hysterical façade. The readiness, moreover, with which such patients develop intense transference feelings may effectively disguise the more basic developmental failure which impairs their capacity for therapeutic alliance. Some patients originally diagnosed as classical hysterics are found to fall within this developmental pattern as their treatment proceeds. Many of them are not capable of maintaining a sufficiently stable therapeutic alliance to tolerate the interpretation of the transference neurosis. While the appropriate therapy for those patients who are not suitable for psychoanalysis is not germane to this discussion, the problems which they present are nevertheless familiar in less severe forms during the course of analysis of every patient. We must recognize that even the most analysable patients will have some defences and some developmental vulnerabilities similar to those shown in more serious disorders. Healthy basic equipment is never absolutely prophylactic against partial ego regression leading to diminishing self-esteem or transient impairment of reality testing. Although such threatened regression of the autonomous ego may be expressed by current anxieties, it nevertheless derives from very primitive sources.

These primitive sources illustrate the suggestions relevant to association between the object relations and ego identification with which I opened this chapter. It is too often assumed that references to the primitive source of the doctor–patient relationship in psychoanalysis imply that the analytic situation represents a repetition of the early mother–child relationship. Such assumptions have stimulated strong objections on the part of those who, following Richard Sterba (1934) and Edward Bibring (1953), stress the mature features of that part of the patient's ego which allies itself with the analyst. A differentiation must, however, be made between theoretical understanding of a developmental origin and the technique appropriate in the analytic situation. Such differentiation is in keeping with Hartmann's emphasis on the need to expand our understanding of the developmental aspects of different ego functions.

In brief, I would propose that psychoanalytic treatment may be compared with the forward-moving developmental model here illustrated, with certain important modifications. The initial stages of analysis, which involve the establishment of a therapeutic alliance, seldom fail to elicit some primitive objective anxiety which may be differentiated from the specific content of the transference neurosis. Although this anxiety is subject to considerable individual variation, the initial stage, in essence, involves achievement of a new and special object relationship in a two-person situation. This initiates a new ego identification which, it is proposed, determines the nature, quality and stability of the therapeutic alliance, which may thus be defined as both an object relationship and an ego identification.

I have suggested as a major premise of this discussion that the first and most significant object relationship leading to an ego identification occurs in the early mother–child relationship. The nature and quality of this early achievement can be correlated with the initiation of secondary ego autonomy. This, as shown in the model, is to be regarded as the core of that part of basic ego equipment which remains most consistent throughout individual life. The analytic situation as a one-to-one relationship will inevitably draw on the strengths and reveal the weaknesses determined by the initial achievement. The significance of object relations in determining certain ego attributes not only applies to their initiation; it is equally necessary for their maintenance, particularly in stressful one-to-one relationships.

Relevant to this discussion is Ernst Kris's suggestion relating early ego identification to the mother's adaptation to the child's innate potentialities in the period preceding self-object differentiation. As I suggested earlier, 'The role of the analyst in the opening phases of treatment should here be compared and contrasted.... the analytic situation demands from the outset maximal mobilization of those ego attributes which remain for the most part contingent on the success achieved at a relatively early stage of psychic development. Such mobilization will be fostered by intuitive adaptive responses on the part of the analyst which may well be compared to those of the successful parent... In brief, the analyst in the opening stages of treatment helps the patient to integrate within the analytic relationship ego capacities which had previously been successful in areas outside the sphere of neurotic conflict.'

This feature of the analytic situation has often been noted in respect of both the opening and terminal stages of analysis. It must be emphasized, however, that no patient will be capable of tolerating the added stress aroused by the emergence of the transference neurosis unless the therapeutic alliance is not only established but maintained at all times. We may here see another analogy to the original developmental process. To paraphrase, it is only the child who has established an early positive ego identification who can maintain positive object relations and added ego identifications during the vicissitudes of later periods of childhood development culminating in the triangular oedipal situation. Neurotic symptoms or character traits will, in such cases, mainly derive from intrapsychic defences mobilized by anxiety as the signal of internal danger. Transference analysis in such cases involves the reopening of conflicts previously closed off by neurotic excessive or inadequate defences, aiming towards the goal of a more adaptive resolution. This, however, is contingent on the maintenance and progressive integration of secure object relations, i.e. the therapeutic alliance.

The analyst must of course remain objective and dispassionate during the interpretation of fantasies and wishes derived from the repressed, forgotten past. In this role he resembles the parent who can recognize without gratifying the child's oedipal fantasies during the infantile neurosis. He must, at the same time, ally himself with the patient, remaining an object for continued positive ego identification. His role is thus by no means confined to interpretation of the transference neurosis. Of special importance in this context is the consistent mutual recognition that passive acceptance of the inevitable is just as basic to psychic maturity as active responses and adaptive mastery in available areas of gratification and achievement.

To return to our figure, the analytical process involves in essence the revival in the new setting of the analytic situation of that which was previously experienced during the period between self-object differentiation and the childhood crossing of the two reciprocal curves. This implies that preceding experience (i.e. before self-object differentiation), although of the utmost importance in determining crucial ego attributes, is not in general subject to substantial modification in a traditional psychoanalysis. Such ego attributes cannot, however, be taken for granted. They must be maintained and strengthened as the analysis proceeds. The analyst must respond at all times to affect which indicates the patient's need to feel respected and acknowledged as a real person. As the transference neurosis develops, however, significant regression in the two reciprocal curves is an essential concomitant. As this occurs, the analyst becomes increasingly significant as a displaced object in respect of unresolved unconscious infantile conflict.

Successful analysis thus demands a dual approach to the therapeutic process. This highlights the intimate relationship and the crucial differences between the transference neurosis which is subject to infinite changeability, and the therapeutic alliance, which as a real relationship requires a consistent, stable nucleus. Such a dual approach implies a developmental differentiation between the defensive ego which must regress, and the autonomous ego which must retain the capacity for consistent object relations.

It must also be recognized, however, that the earliest ego identifications, although of the utmost significance, initiate rather than actually determine all that is included in the autonomous ego and the self concept. Later stages of infantile development thus influence both positively and negatively the availability of earliest achievement. Although substantial early success is to be regarded as relatively irreversible, later identifications are subject to many vicissitudes throughout the development and resolution of the infantile neurosis. These identifications may be destined for later incorporation in the autonomous ego, the defensive ego, and/or the superego and ego-ideal. Their definitive locality thus influences not only the sense of personal identity but also the areas of prohibited and permitted instinctual activity, both sexualized and non-sexualized. The analytic process should not only alter the perception of internal danger but should also bring about progressive modification of those ego and superego identifications which had previously stimulated neurotic ego defences. As this occurs, concurrent changes take place both in the content of transference material and in the quality and stability of the therapeutic alliance.

Such changes, during the course of successful transference analysis, determine important differences between the opening and the terminal phases of treatment. The similarities in the reappearance of primitive fantasies and separation anxiety are too well known to require detailed comment. Their appearance highlights the regressive concomitants of all maturational crises. Whereas, however, the opening phases serve to initiate the passive components of a prolonged developmental process, termination represents a move towards significant autonomy and independence. The degree of passivity and dependence required for the analytic process represents an increasingly ego-alien wish as termination approaches. Though the analyst must interpret primitive dependent wishes as they recur, he is no longer in a position comparable to a parent responding to the early developmental process. The patient must now achieve a mature acceptance of realistic limitations consistent with active motivation towards autonomy and independence. The analyst as an object for continued positive ego identification must be retained within the area of autonomous ego functions. He must also remain a potentially available object in case of future need. No patient, in short, reaches successful termination of analysis unless he recognizes that he is not so invulnerable that he could not return for advice or help if need arose.

Termination of psychoanalysis thus implies a mature acceptance of limitations in respect, first, of analysis and the analyst; second, the patient's optimal capacities for future achievement; and finally, the degree of gratification which may be anticipated from reality itself. It is hardly surprising that this complex task should involve anxiety, depression and regressive wishes. The analyst is now, however, in a position comparable to that of the parent who accepts and fosters the growing independence of his child. Termination of analysis is thus not confined to the reclosure already indicated. It also involves interpretation and integration of those passive components of the therapeutic alliance which facilitate future regression in the service of the ego. Termination thus resembles successful mourning in that the analyst, as a continued supportive parental surrogate, is on the whole renounced. While such forthcoming renunciation mobilizes affect which contains components of both anxiety and depression, successful mastery will substantially increase future autonomy and freedom.

To summarize, let me reiterate my earlier statements regarding the significance of intrapsychic conflict and its resolution in the theory of the psychoanalytic process. Psychoanalytic treatment presents many analogies to the early developmental process.

First, successful development in the later stages of infancy is contingent on the earlier establishment of good object relationships which must be maintained. As a corollary, successful emergence and resolution of the transference neurosis in clinical psychoanalysis is contingent on the establishment and maintenance of the therapeutic alliance. The qualities, moreover, in the analyst which best foster the therapeutic alliance correspond in many ways to those intuitive responses in the mother which lead to successful early ego development in the baby.

Second, psychic development implies at all stages both progressive and regressive manifestations. Regression is thus an inevitable concomitant of forward progressive movement. Such regression can lead to mastery and added adaptation only if basic functions of the ego are maintained. This applies to the infantile neurosis, adolescence, and other developmental crises. It is central to the developmental implications of controlled regression during the analytic process.

Finally, just as healthy development through childhood and adolescence leads to independence, maturity and significant autonomy in the young adult, so too satisfactory termination of a successful analysis also involves autonomy and independence. Both normal maturation and clinical psychoanalysis demand a process of separation which includes components of grief and mourning, leading to the reintegration of successful, stable ego identifications. Neither maturity nor successful analysis, however, can be regarded as an absolute achievement. A crucial capacity for both includes the acceptance of realistic limitations, the renunciation of omnipotent fantasies, and the ability to seek help or support when needed. In this sense, no psychoanalysis should be regarded as conclusively terminated, however successful its outcome may be.

16

PSYCHOANALYSIS AND PSYCHIC HEALTH

In the concluding chapter of the first section of this volume I discussed the relevance of psychoanalysis as a comprehensive developmental psychology to psychiatric evaluation and psychiatric treatment. In this context I discussed the need to understand the role of mental health programmes and different methods of therapeutic intervention in relation to certain crucial landmarks in individual growth and development. Equally important at a time when community psychiatry has become increasingly popular is the need to formulate certain criteria for genuine psychic health. This problem can only be approached through increased understanding of individual psychic structure and function. The contemporary psychoanalyst, from his intensive experience in the treatment of potentially healthy adult patients, should find himself in a position to make important contributions in this area. In this chapter, therefore, I will attempt to extrapolate from both clinical experience and theoretical knowledge a psychoanalytic conception of psychic health. This should be compatible, first, with our current metapsychological assumptions, and in addition with our increasing awareness of the significance for later health or psychopathology of the crucial early years of individual development.

Psychoanalysts have long recognized the fact that external adaptation, however important, need not imply either successful development or immunity from serious underlying psychopathology. Over fifty years ago, for example, Wilfred Trotter emphasized the dangers to psychoanalysis of confusing normal behaviour with healthy psychology.

> Psycho-analytic psychology has grown up under conditions which may very well have encouraged the persistence of the human point of view. . . . The objective standard . . . by which the society was judged was necessarily that of the physician, namely the capacity to restore

the abnormal mind to the 'normal'. Normal in this sense is of course no more than a statistical expression implying the condition of the average man. It could scarcely fail, however, to acquire the significance of 'healthy'. If once the statistically normal mind is accepted as being synonymous with the psychologically healthy mind . . . a standard is set up which has a most fallacious appearance of objectivity (1916, pp. 78–9).

Ernest Jones indicated that 'so-called normality represents a much more devious and obscure way of dealing with the fundamentals of life than the neuroses do, and it is a correspondingly much more difficult route to retrace' (1930, p. 366). In his paper 'The Concept of a Normal Mind' Ernest Jones referred to the opportunities afforded by the analyses of apparently normal candidates. 'In work of this kind', he stated, 'one is often astonished to observe how a comparatively good functioning of the personality can exist with an extensive neurosis, or even psychosis, that is not manifest' (1932, p. 207). These early observations have been amply confirmed by Gitelson, Tartakoff and many others in the much greater experience which has accumulated as a result of years of psychoanalytic popularity after the end of World War II.

In a monograph entitled *Current Concepts of Positive Mental Health* Marie Jahoda (1958) reviewed the literature on the subject. Her introductory remarks are highly relevant to my own thesis:

> One has the option of defining mental health in at least one of two ways: as a relatively constant and enduring function of personality . . . or as a momentary function of personality and situation. Looking at mental health in the first way will lead to a classification of individuals as more or less healthy. Looking at it in the second way will lead to a classification of actions as more or less healthy.

This statement may be illustrated by reference to the clinical experiences during World War II which stimulated my first theoretical paper 'Anxiety and the Capacity to Bear It' (see Chapter 3). Soldiers with a previous history of manifest anxiety proved more resilient after a period of severe stress than many whose history bore substantial evidence of apparent health and successful external adaptation. This finding confirms Edward

Glover's suggestion that 'a normal person must show some capacity for anxiety tolerance' (1932, p. 249). In addition, however, it serves to illustrate Marie Jahoda's distinction between healthy people and healthy actions. An examination of the previous actions of those who reconstituted rapidly often showed that, despite considerable achievements and emotional maturity, they had been somewhat handicapped by phobic–counterphobic character traits, symptoms, inhibitions, or their manifest anxiety. Conversely, the actions, i.e. external adaptation, of the more serious war neurotics had typically been, up to the time of their traumatic experiences, healthy, adjusted and substantially successful. Such individuals, it may be suggested, are unlikely to come to the attention of the psychiatrist or the psychoanalyst until their successful adaptation has, for whatever reasons, been seriously undermined.

One important exception to this statement concerns the problems presented by apparently normal candidates and others who seek personal analysis ostensibly for professional reasons. It is the task of the analyst to explain their good external adaptation in relation to its genesis in childhood development. It is equally important, however, to distinguish the syndrome described as so-called normality from genuine psychic health (which, it may be suggested, includes the capacity for emotional growth). I will attempt to pinpoint the developmental tasks which I believe to be crucial to the individual who will acquire substantial autonomy, a sexualized identity, the capacity for meaningful relations with others and, finally, the capacity for continued emotional growth. My discussion is, however, necessarily confined to individuals living within our own social structure. I am willing to concede the possibility that the kind of adaptation which leads to so-called normality in our own culture might be adequate for the achievement of adaptation and acceptable psychic health in societies which provide the type of social structure which does not demand what we regard as autonomy. It may also occur in those societies in which the capacity for a definitive heterosexual object choice is not considered to be an integral feature of emotional maturity.

As Dr. Jahoda suggested, the problems of defining psychic health, or normality, are closely related to our understanding of character and its development. At the mid-winter meeting of the American Psychoanalytic Association in 1957 Dr. Helen Tartakoff chaired a panel on 'The Psychoanalytic Concept of Character'. In her introductory remarks she reviewed the literature on the subject, concluding, according to the published report:

> Complex genetic and dynamic factors are involved whether the conflicts be solved by reality-adjusted, well-integrated behavior leading to apparent normality or, in contrast, whether a neurotic compromise results, producing overt symptomatology or a character neurosis (Tartakoff, 1958, p. 567).

The clinical material presented at this panel proves retrospectively highly relevant to the thesis of this chapter. Samuel Atkin (1958) presented material derived from the analyses of several apparently well-adjusted persons, in effect so-called normal. When, however, he began to look beneath the surface he was impressed by, among other things, 'a prominence of primitive ego defences'.

In some contrast, during the same panel discussion Annie Reich (1958) presented her analysis of another patient, also 'considered by both himself and his environment as normal'. It should be noted, however, that this patient spontaneously sought analysis because of his own subjective awareness of restrictions in his work productivity. In his case, also, an apparently healthy façade covered serious inhibitions and a serious neurosis. His analysis, however, was substantially successful, far more than those described by Dr. Atkin, who had explicitly referred to a 'relatively rigid and unalterable residue'.

In his discussion of this paper Maxwell Gitelson (1958*b*) referred to some of the criteria of psychic health. With reference to Annie Reich's case, he suggested that 'the earliest relationship between mother and child was of great importance for future development'. Concluding the discussion, Atkin commented that he too felt that an early satisfactory identification must have been the factor accounting for the excellent functioning and maturity of Annie Reich's patient. Since it is relevant to certain aspects of my own thesis, it is worth repeating that this patient, even before the analysis, was subjectively aware of internal problems which were limiting, though not preventing, overtly successful external adaptation.

Symptom formation and character formation was a central subject of discussion at the International Congress of Psychoanalysis held at Stockholm in 1963. Two papers by Jeanne Lampl-de Groot (1963) and Jacob Arlow (1963) were published in the *International Journal of Psycho-Analysis* before the meeting. In my prepared discussion of these papers I made a differentiation between character development and symptom formation compatible with Marie Jahoda's distinction between healthy and unhealthy individuals and healthy or unhealthy actions.

It is a cardinal feature of psychic life that every important maturational challenge presents highly significant regressive threats. . . . A wide range of functions relevant to definitive personality structure are established at different periods of developmental change. . . . Character formation thus includes the whole range of solutions, adaptive or maladaptive, to recognized developmental challenges. Symptom formation, in contrast, though inevitable during certain maturational crises, is not to be defined as a progressive, but as a regressive phenomenon. It occurs as a result of impairment . . . in the capacity of the psychic apparatus to deal adaptively with the external and/or internal stimuli to which it is exposed. Such impairment, whether acute or chronic, may be brought about by the widest variety of precipitating events (Zetzel, 1964, p. 153).

This definition permits us to include manifest affective distress during recognized developmental or situational crises within the range of potentially healthy psychological structure and function. It implies in addition that limited symptomatology attributable to partial failures in the resolution of specific intrapsychic conflicts may be seen in individuals whose potential for genuine maturity is greater than that of individuals who have consolidated primitive or regressive defences in their definitive character structure. I suggested, however, that both papers revealed an area of significant difficulty in our understanding of psychic health and psychopathology. Both authors emphasized the importance of pre-oedipal experience for the development of healthy and pathological character structure.

Studies of infancy and the earlier years have . . . increasingly stressed the impact of pre-oedipal experience on ego development. Relative success or failure in the establishment of genuine object relations and early ego identification influences both the predisposition to serious disorder and the development and mastery of the infantile neurosis (Zetzel, 1964, p. 151).

The fact that symptoms or character traits attributable to early (pre-oedipal) developmental failure might be differentiated from character traits or symptoms established at a later, i.e. oedipal, level was thus implicitly acknowledged. The discussion of symptom formation was nevertheless in general limited to the neuroses. Neurotic symptoms were thus defined as responses to signal anxiety as described by Freud in 'Inhibitions, Symptoms and Anxiety' (1926). As Arlow, for example, emphasized, however, this type of anxiety is only established at a relatively late stage of childhood development. Both papers suggested, in summary, that our theory had not as yet clearly conceptualized the meeting point and the overlap between pregenital experience and the infantile neurosis. It is a primary goal of this chapter to approach this very difficult area in the light of our contemporary expanded developmental hypothesis.

Certain suggestions put forward by Ives Hendrick (1942, 1943, 1951) are relevant to my own approach to this subject. His emphasis in several papers on the child's spontaneous efforts towards mastery are in keeping with my own understanding of affect tolerance and mastery. Whether or not one postulates a basic instinct in this context is, I believe, less important than recognition of motivation towards mastery as an integral component of both external and internal adaptation. In addition, Hendrick's emphasis on the importance of differentiating mastery of ambivalence in one-to-one (dyadic) relations from the more complex tasks posed by the emergence of a triangular (i.e. triadic) conflict is, I believe, crucial to our understanding of those attributes of psychic health and psychopathology which derive from relative success or failure regarding these very different developmental challenges.

In my own approach I have somewhat expanded Hendrick's conception of dyadic relationships. Mastery of ambivalence in the early mother–child relationship remains, in my opinion, prerequisite to optimal future mental health. Relative failures in this area may be consistent with long periods of successful external adaptation. However, serious regressive responses to later developmental crises—adolescence, marriage, parenthood, retirement and old age—typically reveal significant failures in this original developmental task. In addition, clinical experience has led me to the conclusion that successful pre-oedipal development involves the establishment of more than one essentially dyadic relationship. In brief, the child who will later become a potentially healthy adult has established successful one-to-one relationships with both parents before the onset of the genital oedipal triangular situation. Under these circumstances genuine intrapsychic conflict fosters the capacity to differentiate between external and internal reality. This I believe is an indispensable attribute of the healthy or potentially healthy (analysable neurotic) individual.

In a recent paper entitled 'Character Formation in Adolescence' (1968) Peter Blos suggests that the regression so characteristic of this period of life facilitates the definitive achievement of four developmental tasks. These he defines as the second individuation, achievement of ego continuity, integration of a sexual identity, and mastery of residual trauma. I believe that our understanding of these various tasks may be increased by a distinction between the instinctual regression which reopens otherwise defended-against intrapsychic conflict and regression of the ego to the pregenital period of one-to-one relationships. It may thus be suggested that Dr. Blos's first two developmental tasks, second individuation and the achievement of ego continuity, mainly involve a definitive integration of capacities initiated during the first process of individuation. This, according to Margaret Mahler (1963, 1965, 1969), takes place during the second and third years of life. As I will amplify somewhat later, it may also be suggested that the achievement of a sexual identity and mastery of residual trauma derive from the more complex tasks posed by the emergence of a triangular or oedipal conflict.

I will first amplify my own understanding of the first two developmental tasks discussed by Peter Blos. I have elsewhere suggested that these tasks are not confined to the process of individuation (Zetzel, 1964). They also include initiation of the capacity to recognize, tolerate and master painful affect. Mastery of ambivalence is prerequisite to success in both the first and second periods of individuation. Recognition, tolerance and mastery of both anxiety and depression, defined by Edward Bibring (1953) as basic ego states, are to be regarded as equally indispensable. I have mentioned these steps in the order in which I myself became aware of them. I would now like to raise a question, however, as to whether I was correct in my initial impression that this represents the order of explicit chronological development. Rather, there is much to suggest that major progress is mainly limited during infancy, the childhood neurosis and latency to the last developmental task, i.e. all that is involved in mastery—namely learning, achievement and some façade of independence. This is compatible with the mere beginnings, i.e. very initial steps, regarding the recognition and tolerance of depression and anxiety as integral features of the affective position which I believe must precede genuine mastery of separation and narcissistic injury. In so far, however, as depression and its tolerance and its mastery are to be regarded as necessary components of psychic health, I would agree with Dr. Blos that this represents a crucial feature of the second period of individuation which is closely related to his second developmental task, achievement of ego continuity. It may also be suggested that the capacity to establish a successful therapeutic alliance in adult analysis is significantly determined by the degree to which this second process of individuation resulted in the capacity to tolerate anxiety, depression and intrapsychic conflict.

I would like to suggest that the type of so-called normality which is compatible with serious underlying pathology typically develops in individuals who have substantially failed in certain aspects of these early developmental tasks. Like the syndrome I have elsewhere described as so-called good hysteria (Chapter 14), the so-called normal individual has substantially failed during the pre-oedipal period to recognize or to tolerate either anxiety or depression. His major defences are not directed against ego-alien fantasies and wishes. They are rather still motivated by the more primitive wish to obtain and retain external approval, i.e. narcissistic supplies. It is often the case that such individuals have achieved adequate primary ego autonomy and, in addition, may be naturally gifted regarding the tasks imposed by the environment. External adaptation may thus be consistent for a long period of time with emotional immaturity, shallow object relations and conformity with the ideals of a particular environment.

In a recent paper entitled 'The Normal Personality in our Culture and the Nobel Prize Complex' (1966) Helen Tartakoff emphasized the degree to which the 'success goals fostered in our culture' lead to character-defensive behaviour which serves adaptive purposes. She further expanded Maxwell Gitelson's earlier discussion (1958*b*) of the problems incurred in the analyses of so-called normal candidates. She suggested in conclusion:

> In this child-centred culture the mother-child interactions which occur before true causality has been established, have a number of potential consequences . . . [that] may lay the foundation for the child's expectation of receiving recognition and reward for his adaptive achievements. They tend to perpetuate derivatives of omnipotence in the form of narcissistic fantasies (1966, p. 249).

My own thesis is somewhat different, though not incompatible with Dr. Tartakoff's. I have already suggested that emotional maturity requires the capacity to recognize, tolerate and master painful affect (e.g. anxiety and depression). Unless the initial steps had been made during the pre-oedipal years, continued active adaptation may, as Dr. Tartakoff suggests, imply omnipotent fantasies, narcissistic goals and significant failure to accept either one's own limitations or the limitations of reality. I would agree that a culture which places excessive premium on success may prolong and reinforce such developmental failures. At the same time, however, I personally doubt that any early mother–child relationships can be so totally rewarding that the child has no opportunity to recognize and experience relative helplessness, separation anxiety or some awareness of his own limitations. I would therefore tend to attribute this form of so-called normality to developmental failure regarding the developmental tasks I have outlined in respect of the first period of individuation.

In the same paper Dr. Tartakoff concluded: 'This narcissistic orientation complicates the establishment of object relations and the resolution of the oedipal conflict' (1966, p. 249). I would be inclined to emphasize this point even more strongly. Indeed, I would suggest that significant failures in mastery of ambivalence in one-to-one relations may not only complicate but substantially impair the emergence, let alone the resolution, of a genuine triangular oedipal conflict. Initiation, it may be suggested, of the capacity to recognize, tolerate and master affective distress takes place in healthy development in the context of one-to-one relations. It is important that such relations should be established with both parents before the onset of the genital oedipal period. Each parent, in other words, will have been experienced both as a love object and as an object for identification during the pre-oedipal years. The mother is usually the first object with whom an ego identification is made. In optimal development, however, the child adds during the pre-oedipal years both an object relation and some degree of identification with the father. In the boy this identification is a precursor of the man's sense of masculine identity. In the girl such an identification may, on the one hand, be motivated by a relationship with the father less ambivalent than that achieved with the mother. It is also, however, a frequent concomitant of the defensive reinforcement of penis envy which is typically encountered in the analysis of potentially healthy women who may or may not suffer from a circumscribed hysterical transference neurosis. (See Chapter 14.)

I have discussed in some detail both the progressive and the regressive aspects of challenges which may be considered in the context of one-to-one relations. Such challenges first arise during the pre-oedipal years and are typically re-experienced during adolescence. The achievement and maintenance of adult autonomy are never, however, to be regarded as fixed or unalterable. Clinical experience in the analysis of neurotic patients clearly reveals important progressive modifications in this area during the course and termination of a successful therapeutic analysis. Related challenges may also be recognized in respect of many other periods of developmental change throughout the life cycle. Such challenges must, however, be clearly distinguished from the more complex internalizations which I believe originate during the child's experience of a genuine triangular oedipal situation. Success or failure in these initial developmental tasks is particularly relevant to individual responses to the real losses and restrictions which must be anticipated in the later years of life. To quote:

> Brief, simple depressive episodes might be regarded as inevitable concomitants of the wide variety of renunications which must be accepted in the later years of life. . . . The ageing inividual who responds with transient, reversible simple depression is repeating in essence a process of accepting both his own and the world's limitations which began in early childhood. Such acceptance need not result in resignation or despair. It may indeed facilitate new adaptations appropriate to the achievements and gratifications which still remain available. . . . The inner resources [which make this possible] were first acquired early in life. Insofar as they have been genuinely achieved, they remain potentially available at every later developmental crisis. In this sense, [every period of life] can, as Erik Erikson (1950) suggested, be included within the framework of a comprehensive developmental psychology (Zetzel, 1965, pp. 115, 119).

In summary, Dr. Blos's first two developmental tasks may be considered in the context of one-to-one relations. These tasks clearly differ from those presented by the instinctual regression which in essence reopens the more complex conflicts which determined the infantile neurosis. The reopening of a genuine triangular conflict offers the adolescent a second opportunity of resolving this crucial conflict. Success will include as a major goal the achievement of a genuine sexualized identity. For this to occur mastery of residual trauma remains an important prerequisite. The individual who has successfully accomplished all four of Dr. Blos's tasks will not only have achieved genuine individuation and autonomy but will also have integrated a sexual identity sufficiently secure to permit a satisfactory heterosexual object choice. In addition, such individuals will have achieved the capacity to utilize neutralized psychic energy in areas of conflict-free activity.

It is perhaps of some interest to note the curious historical paradox which determines my phraseology. Recognition of the infantile oedipal conflict was one of Freud's early major discoveries. For a long time this conflict and the various anxieties which it entails were regarded as the main determinants of adult neurotic illness. The increased emphasis recently placed on the significance of the pregenital years, however relevant, should not lead us to discount the importance of the oedipal period.

The individual who has experienced a genuine triangular conflict may be regarded as potentially healthy, whether or not the conflict has been fully resolved. I am thus suggesting that a psychoanalytic approach to the criteria of psychic health implicitly includes a differentiation between those individuals who, despite neurotic symptoms, neurotic character traits or manifest anxiety or depression, appear capable of achieving substantial health and those, conversely, who, whatever their overt symptomatology or so-called 'normal' behaviour may be, have failed to pass certain crucial landmarks in the acquisition of potential or actual psychic health. From this point of view I would still maintain that recognition and tolerance of the anxiety integral to the emergence of genuine intrapsychic conflict are essential attributes of psychic health and the sustained capacity for emotional growth.

An analytic discussion of this topic is complicated by the fact that our major source of detailed information must derive from our knowledge of individuals who have successfully undergone a personal analysis. From this knowledge we may be able to extrapolate certain criteria which would enable us to decide whether 'normal' behaviour and adjustment fall into the category of so-called normal, i.e. reflects serious developmental failure, or whether we accept the behaviour and adjustment of certain individuals as genuinely healthy even though they may not have sought a personal analysis. Both individuals should, in other words, fall into the category of analysable patients, whether or not this treatment is indicated.

In my own clinical experience I have not found that all the apparently well-adjusted individuals who have sought analysis for professional reasons fall into the group of disturbed, so-called normals. Many of them, although quite well adjusted to a degree comparable with that described by Annie Reich, are aware of constriction, inhibition or anxiety in either their careers or their relations with others. These individuals demonstrate during the course of their analysis both hysterical and obsessional mechanisms. In general, the most analysable women in this group have shown some hysterical symptoms and/or character traits, usually in their heterosexual object relations. They have also shown some obsessional defences. The most analysable men have also demonstrated during the course of analysis partial failure in their resolution of the oedipal situation. Like Dr. Reich's patient, however, their presenting problems are usually obsessional and/or inhibitory rather than overtly hysterical. Many of them, despite a successful work history, have experienced problems in reaching their full potential. In attempting to explain this sexual differentiation, I come to another area of crucial importance in formulating a psychoanalytic approach to psychic health. This question concerns the relationship between activity and passivity in mental life.

Understanding of this question implies a conceptual differentiation between clearly sexualized aspects of activity and passivity and ego attributes, including energy available in areas of conflict-free activity which does not necessarily derive entirely from the libidinal (i.e. sexual) instincts. Libidinal wishes and activities at the genital level are of course subject to an obvious sexual differentiation. Man's typical sexual gratification is reached through active genitality. Mature genital femininity requires the capacity for passive acceptance of another person's (the man's) activity as the major source of sexual gratification. It is readily understandable that men frequently tend to equate activity with masculinity. Women, conversely, often tend to regard femininity as essentially passive. As I have indicated, however, mastery of ambivalence in one-to-one relationships is a crucial early landmark. Such ambivalence clearly implies not only libidinal but also hostile aggressive impulses towards an object seen as both gratifying and frustrating. In optimal development I have suggested that the individual is able during the original developmental process to initiate both passive acceptance and active mastery regarding the conflicts, frustrations and separations of early life. Such initiation includes the capacity to modify and modulate feelings of anger in the process of mobilizing active impulses regarding available goals and ideals. Such active mastery is a necessary prerequisite for later mental health, whatever the sex of the individual.

When, therefore, we consider the role of activity and passivity in the ego's recognition, tolerance and mastery of ambivalence, anxiety and depression, a sharp sexual differentiation should not be made. Psychic health demands successful initiation and later integration of those capacitities which will facilitate throughout life, first, passive recognition and tolerance of limitations, losses and threats, and equally, active efforts towards finding and obtaining available objects and personal goals which permit both passive gratification and active achievement. It may, however, be suggested that the areas of relative developmental failure typically encountered in potentially healthy men and women are subject to a sexual differentiation. It is, in brief, easier and more ego-syntonic for the man to mobilize active resources and related defences than it is passively to experience and tolerate anxiety, depression and delay. In women, conversely, the more typical relative developmental failures derive from problems relevant to ego modes of mastery. At one extreme, certain women, namely those whose penis envy is excessive or defensively reinforced, may have problems in achieving mature femininity. At the other extreme, those women who overemphasize the passive components of femininity may show relative failure in the areas of active mastery.

Understanding of this difference poses many difficult problems. It is clear, for example, that healthy little girls, during the pre-oedipal years, usually demonstrate a considerable degree of independence and activity. I have discussed in another chapter the positive value for future psychic health of the early initiation of these active capacities. Peter Blos's suggestion that it is only in adolescence that a genuine sexual identification is integrated opens the possibility that many factors, both external and internal, may determine the nature and stability of both male and female ego-ideals. In so far as men can equate masculinity with continued active striving they may sacrifice to a significant degree the passive components of maturity. These, it may be suggested, are integral to the capacity to regress in the service of the ego and also to the creative process. It is important that defensive overmobilization of activity as a result of adolescent development should be distinguished from initial developmental failure. The former is not incompatible with potential psychic health; the latter is often concomitant to the so-called normality which has already been discussed. Conversely, in so far as women, particularly during adolescence, equate femininity with passivity, only permitting activity in purely domestic functions, a parallel sacrifice has been made. Provided, however, that the original developmental tasks have been successfully accomplished, many women prove in later years capable of remobilizing their active capacities, thus finding areas for individual gratification.

The mature creative man does not rely entirely on continued active achievement in order to maintain his self-esteem. He is also capable of some contemplation, outside interests and participation in activities which do not demand continued evidence of success. He has usually at some time in his life gone through an experience of disappointment, loss or sadness. He has certainly experienced the affect of anxiety in some form at some time. He has also, however, been able to work through his incestuous rivalry. He can thus differentiate active competition regarding available goals from competition in the oedipal rivalry situation. Relative failure in this latter area is, I believe, one of the reasons why the presenting complaint of so many analysable men concerns problems of professional achievement. Successful development and/or successful analysis of the potentially healthy man will permit mobilization of active resources without excluding the passive component of maturity.

The most mature woman, conversely, does not rely entirely on external objects as the source of gratification and pleasure. She has also achieved personal areas of active gratification and mastery. The healthy or successfully analysed woman should be able to combine successful marriage and motherhood with some sort of personal career. Her investment in this career is usually secondary to her investment in her home and family during the years of her children's maturation. She can, however, renew and reinforce her previous activities as her children grow up. Relative failures in this area may not be evident in many married women until quite late in life. It is only during the ageing process that earlier developmental failures may become evident in both sexes. The individual who has substantially succeeded in the initiation of the major attributes of psychic maturity is, I believe, unlikely to regress in a significant or irreversible manner when confronted with the realistic changes posed during the ageing process. This would imply that our criteria of psychic health must be considered in a developmental context. It would also appear impossible to present any absolute psychoanalytic criteria of psychic health. I have suggested, however, that a relative approach will emphasize certain crucial developmental landmarks as determinants of the definitive capacity to achieve or to regain psychic health.

I have already suggested that not all individuals who meet the accepted criteria for normal behaviour confirm in the analytic situation the suggestion that external adaptation is necessarily incompatible with substantial success in respect of these developmental landmarks. The analysis of such individuals has, however, amply confirmed the crucial importance of the infantile oedipal situation, both as a prerequisite for mental health and as a continued unresolved conflict in the potentially healthy, analysable neurotic. In my own experience, both as an analyst and as a supervisor, the analysis of such patients has confirmed their early favourable development regarding the initiation of what I have described as essential prerequisites to adult psychological health. In the large majority of analysable neurotic patients, however, the analysis has revealed adverse experiences either during the infantile neurosis itself or early in the post-oedipal years. Such adverse experiences include a wide range from, at one extreme, permanent loss of one or other parent through death to, at the other, some impairment of the mother–child relationship following the birth of a younger sibling at a crucial period of the patient's development. In essence such experiences have tended to undermine one or other of the pre-oedipal one-to-one relationships, thus impairing the child's capacity to tolerate, let alone to master, the internal struggles of this crucial period. In a number of patients falling within this group there had, in addition, been a period of prolonged exposure to the primal scene.

Our understanding of trauma and its impact on both character formation and the predisposition to neurosis must be determined in part by our understanding of the repetition compulsion. Dr. Blos's fourth developmental task, mastery of residual trauma, clearly implies that potentially healthy and adaptive growth includes the compulsion to revive and repeat traumatic experiences. The repetition compulsion is at least in part attributable to the positive wish to master. Such mastery includes not only the effects of painful stimulation from the external world; it also includes tolerance and mastery of the anxiety which was aroused through a process of gradual internalization. It involves, finally, tolerance and mastery of the helplessness, namely the depressive affect, which had been felt at the time of the traumatic experience by a related process. From analysis, as well as psychiatric and psychotherapeutic experience, I have come to the conclusion that it is not only the severity but even more the chronology of traumatic experiences which influences the degree to which the repetition is motivated by the wish to master and internalize. Since serious trauma very early in life may interfere with the basic attributes of psychic health, they are outside the scope of this discussion. I believe, however, that the type of traumatic experience which occurs during or after the emergence of a triangular oedipal situation is consistent with the later achievement of substantial psychic health. In the most favourable cases it is arguable that the years of adolescence will facilitate the spontaneous resolution of this crucial triangle. A number of individuals appear to respond well to relatively brief psychotherapy during the later years of adolescence. The best and most analysable patients, whatever their presenting symptomatology or conversely the lack of it, in my experience fall within this group.

I have suggested that psychic health requires the initiation, during the first years of childhood development, of certain crucial attributes which may be described in terms of our metapsychological premises. These may be summarized briefly. It is during the pre-oedipal years that the maturing child's psychic apparatus acquires structural attributes to cope with dynamic energy which is characterized by economic features. I have explicitly suggested elsewhere that whatever native instinctual endowment may be, the quality of early experience has a decisive influence on the amount and distribution of positive and negative impulses (e.g. aggression and libido) with which the child enters later developmental periods. During this same period psychic structure will develop by a maturational process which, as Freud himself suggested in 'Analysis Terminable and Interminable' (1937), may be partially determined by innate constitutional factors. In addition, however, the quality of the relationships which determine the first ego identifications not only influences later ego development but is also closely related to the internalization of the precursors of the definitive superego. The adaptive capacities of the successfully developing child are first mainly directed towards mastery of external reality. The onset of the infantile oedipal situation results in optimal development in the differentiation between internal and external reality which leads to the emergence of anxiety as the signal for intrapsychic defence. Thus by the time the potentially healthy child reaches this level one may clearly discern in a developmental context the continued validity of our basic metapsychological assumptions. As already noted, however, our developmental hypothesis includes, by definition, both progressive and regressive potentialities at all times. Both developmental and situational crises thus present both maturational challenges and significant regressive threats.

The terminal phases of analysis surely represent an important maturational challenge. It is also well known that this period during most successful analyses is characterized by significant regressive features. The transient or fleeting reappearance of earlier neurotic symptoms is neither surprising nor disturbing. More important is the re-emergence of earlier conflicts which had characterized one-to-one relationships. The terminal stages of a successful analysis are typically characterized by separation anxiety, sadness and even depression. Such regressive experiences are, however, combined with added pleasure in the expanded areas of conflict-free activity which had been facilitated by the analysis of the transference neurosis. Both the progressive and the regressive implications of maturational change are thus highlighted during this crucial period of treatment. It is here too that the individual becomes fully aware of the fact that there can be no absolute criteria of psychic health. Definitive acceptance of the limitations, both of reality and of the self, thus characterizes the terminal phases of a successful analysis. Such acceptance is a necessary prerequisite to the capacity to recognize and tolerate painful affect as an inevitable subjective experience in the face of threatened or actual disappointment and loss. This tolerance, as already suggested, might be regarded as the basis on which the type of genuine mastery I have described as the active component of maturity is optimally developed. Last but not least, the successfully analysed patient will be able to recognize that the termination of analysis is itself to be regarded as a relative rather than an absolute event. I have thus re-emphasized the importance of the pre-oedipal period for the initiation of certain crucial ego attributes; first, the achievement of good one-to-one object relationships and the internalization of stable ego identifications. During this process the individual first develops an ego capable of experiencing anxiety and depression which, as already suggested, are to be regarded as basic ego states. Their recognition, tolerance and mastery must, however, be repeated and reintegrated in different guises and in different forms during every important period of situational and/or developmental change.

In addition, I have underscored the continued significance of the infantile oedipal situation as a crucial landmark in psychological development. Individuals who have reached this level may be regarded as potentially healthy and capable of emotional growth. Relative failures to resolve this conflict when it first arises may impair the solution of two of the developmental tasks of adolescence noted by Peter Blos, namely the mastery of residual trauma and the achievement of a sexualized identity. Such partial failures characterize those individuals who develop an analysable neurosis in adult life. It is arguable, however, that the instinctual regression integral to adolescence offers a second opportunity for successful resolution. In favourable cases, therefore, individuals may emerge from this identity crisis without significant emotional or characterological problems. I have suggested, finally, that both the regressive and progressive features which characterize the terminal phases of analysis confirm, first, the continued need to re-experience and to reintegrate those basic ego qualities first initiated during the pre-oedipal period. In addition, however, both the mobilization and utilization of energy in areas of conflict-free activity, and the achievement and maintenance of a mature sexualized identity, depend on adequate resolution of a genuine oedipal triangular situation.

I will conclude with a quotation:

> [The] setting-up of the reality principle proved to be a momentous step. . . . In the first place, the new demands made a succession of adaptations necessary in the psychical apparatus, which, owing to our insufficient or uncertain knowledge, we can only detail very cursorily. . . . While the ego goes through its transformation from a pleasure-ego into a reality-ego, the sexual instincts undergo the changes that lead them from their original auto-erotism through various intermediate phases to object-love in the service of procreation. If . . . each step in these two courses of development may become the site of a disposition to later neurotic illness, it is plausible to suppose

> that the form taken by the subsequent illness . . . will depend on the particular phase of the development of the ego and of the libido in which the dispositional inhibition of development has occurred. Thus unexpected significance attaches to the chronological features of the two developments (which have not yet been studied), and to possible variations in their synchronization (Freud, 1911, pp. 219–20).

If we add here the capacity for emotional growth, this statement defines in a nutshell the essential problems confronting us. How far can we in 1970 fill in the areas which had not yet been studied when Freud wrote his 'Formulations on the Two Principles of Mental Functioning' more than half a century ago?

REFERENCES

Abraham, K. (1911). Notes on the psycho-analytical investigation and treatment of manic-depressive insanity and allied conditions. *Selected Papers on Psycho-Analysis*. London: Hogarth Press, 1927.

Abraham, K. (1924). A short study of the development of the libido, viewed in the light of mental disorder. *Ibid.*

Alexander, F. (1925). A metapsychological description of the process of cure. *Int. J. Psycho-Anal.*, **6**.

Alexander, F. (1950). Analysis of the therapeutic factors in psychoanalytic treatment. *Psychoanal. Quart.*, **19**.

Arlow, J. A. (1963). Conflict, regression, and symptom formation. *Int. J. Psycho-Anal.*, **44**.

Atkin, S. (1958). A clinical investigation into the nature of character. Abstracted in panel: The psychoanalytic concept of character (rep. by A. F. Valenstein). *J. Amer. psychoanal. Assoc.*, **6**.

Balint, M. (1952). *Primary Love and Psycho-Analytic Technique*. London: Hogarth Press.

Bibring, E. (1937). Contribution to the symposium on the theory of the therapeutic results of psycho-analysis. *Int. J. Psycho-Anal.*, **18**.

Bibring, E. (1947). The so-called English school of psychoanalysis. *Psychoanal. Quart.*, **16**.

Bibring, E. (1953). The mechanism of depression. In *Affective Disorders*, edited by P. Greenacre. New York: International Universities Press.

Bibring, G. L. (1936). A contribution to the subject of transference resistance. *Int. J. Psycho-Anal.*, **17**.

Blos, P. (1968). Character formation in adolescence. *Psychoanal. Study Child*, **23**.

Bornstein, B. (1949). The analysis of a phobic child: some problems of theory and technique in child analyses. *Psychoanal. Study Child*, **3-4**.

Bowlby, J. (1946). *Forty-Four Juvenile Thieves, Their Characters and Home Life*. London: Baillière, Tindall & Cox.

Brain, W. (1963). The languages of psychiatry. *Brit. J. Psychiat.*, **109**.

Brierley, M. (1951). *Trends in Psycho-Analysis*. London: Hogarth Press.

Deutsch, H. (1929). The genesis of agoraphobia. *Int. J. Psycho-Anal.*, **10**.

Easser, B. R. & Lesser, S. R. (1965). Hysterical personality: a re-evaluation. *Psychoanal. Quart.*, **34**.

Eissler, K. R. (1953). The effect of the structure of the ego on psychoanalytic technique. *J. Amer. psychoanal. Assoc.*, **1**.

Erikson, E. H. (1950). *Childhood and Society*. New York: Norton.

Fairbairn, W. R. D. (1943). The war neuroses: their nature and significance. *Brit. med. J.*, **1**.

Fenichel, O. (1939). The counter-phobic attitude. *Int. J. Psycho-Anal.*, **20**.

Fenichel, O. (1941). *Problems of Psychoanalytic Technique*. New York: Psychoanalytic Quarterly Inc.

Fenichel, O. (1945). *The Psychoanalytic Theory of Neurosis*. New York: Norton.

Flügel, J. C. (1939). The examination as initiation rite and anxiety situation. *Int. J. Psycho-Anal.*, **20**.

Freud, A. (1927). Introduction to the technique of child analysis. *The Psycho-Analytical Treatment of Children*. London: Hogarth Press, 1959; New York: International Universities Press, 1959.

Freud, A. (1936). *The Ego and the Mechanisms of Defence*. London: Hogarth Press, 1937; New York: Int. Univ. Press, 1946.

Freud, A. (1949). Aggression in relation to emotional development: normal and pathological. *Psychoanal. Study Child*, **3-4**.

Freud, A. (1954). The widening scope of indications for psychoanalysis. *J. Amer. psychoanal. Assoc.*, **2**.

Freud, S. (1900). The interpretation of dreams. *Standard Edition of the Complete Psychological Works of Sigmund Freud*, **4-5**.

Freud, S. (1905*a*). On psychotherapy. *Standard Edition*, **7**.

Freud, S. (1905*b*). Fragment of an analysis of a case of hysteria. *Standard Edition*, **7**.

Freud, S. (1905*c*). Three essays on the theory of sexuality. *Standard Edition*, **7**.

Freud, S. (1909*a*). Notes upon a case of obsessional neurosis. *Standard Edition*, **10**.

Freud, S. (1909*b*). Analysis of a phobia in a five-year-old boy. *Standard Edition*, **10**.

Freud, S. (1910). Observations on 'wild' psycho-analysis. *Standard Edition*, **11**.

Freud, S. (1911). Formulations on the two principles of mental functioning. *Standard Edition*, **12**.

Freud, S. (1912). Recommendations to physicians practising psycho-analysis. *Standard Edition*, **12**.

Freud, S. (1913*a*). Further recommendations on the technique of psycho-analysis: on beginning the treatment. *Standard Edition*, **12**.

Freud, S. (1913*b*). The disposition to obsessional neurosis: a contribution to the problem of choice of neurosis. *Standard Edition*, **12**.

Freud, S. (1914). On narcissism: an introduction. *Standard Edition*, **14**.

Freud, S. (1917). Mourning and melancholia. *Standard Edition*, **14**.

Freud, S. (1918). From the history of an infantile neurosis. *Standard Edition*, **17**.

Freud, S. (1920). Beyond the pleasure principle. *Standard Edition*, **18**.

Freud, S. (1926). Inhibitions, symptoms and anxiety. *Standard Edition*, **20**.

Freud, S. (1933). New introductory lectures on psycho-analysis. *Standard Edition*, **22**.

Freud, S. (1937). Analysis terminable and interminable. *Standard Edition*, **23**.

Gerö, G. (1936). The construction of depression. *Int. J. Psycho-Anal.*, **17**.

Gitelson, M. (1958*a*). On ego distortion. *Int. J. Psycho-Anal.*, **39**.

Gitelson, M. (1958*b*). Discussant in panel: The psychoanalytic concept of character (rep. by A. F. Valenstein). *J. Amer. psychoanal. Assoc.*, **6**.

Gitelson, M. (1962). The curative factors in psychoanalysis: the first phase of psychoanalysis. *Int. J. Psycho-Anal.*, **43**.

Glover, E. (1932). Medico-psychological aspects of normality. *On the Early Development of Mind*. London: Imago, 1956; New York: International Universities Press, 1956.

Glover, E. (1942). Notes on the psychological effects of war conditions on the civilian population. III. The 'Blitz'—1940-41. *Int. J. Psycho-Anal.*, **23**.

Glover, E. (1945). Examination of the Klein system of child psychology. *Psychoanal. Study Child*, **1**.

Glover, E. (1947). Basic mental concepts: their clinical and theoretical value. *Psychoanal. Quart.*, **16**.

Glover, E. (1954). Therapeutic criteria of psycho-analysis. *Int. J. Psycho-Anal.*, **35**.

Glover, E. (1955). *The Technique of Psychoanalysis*. New York: International Universities Press.

Greenacre, P. (1941). The predisposition to anxiety. *Trauma, Growth and Personality*. London: Hogarth Press, 1952; New York: International Universities Press, 1969.

Greenacre, P. (1945). The biologic economy of birth. *Ibid.*

Greenacre, P. (1952). *Trauma, Growth and Personality*. London: Hogarth Press; New York: International Universities Press, 1959.

Greenacre, P. (1954). The role of transference: practical considerations in relation to psychoanalytic therapy. *J. Amer. psychoanal. Assoc.*, **2**.

Greenacre, P. (1958). On transference. Abstracted in panel: Technical aspects of transference (rep. by D. Leach). *J. Amer. psychoanal. Assoc.*, **6**.

Greenson, R. R. (1959). Phobia, trauma and the ego. Abstracted in panel: Phobias and their vicissitudes (rep. by L. Ferber). *J. Amer. psychoanal. Assoc.*, **7**.

Greenson, R. R. (1960). Empathy and its vicissitudes. *Int. J. Psycho-Anal.*, **41**.

Hartmann, H. (1939). *Ego Psychology and the Problem of Adaptation*. New York: International Universities Press, 1958.

Hartmann, H. (1950). Psychoanalysis and developmental psychology. *Essays on Ego Psychology*. New York: International Universities Press, 1964.

Hartmann, H. (1951). Technical implications of ego psychology. *Ibid.*

Hartmann, H. (1952). The mutual influences in the development of ego and id. *Ibid.*

Hartmann, H. (1954). Problems of infantile neurosis. *Ibid.*

Hartmann, H. (1964). *Essays on Ego Psychology*. New York: International Universities Press.

Hartmann, H., Kris, E. & Loewenstein, R. M. (1946). Comments on the formation of psychic structure. *Psychoanal. Study Child*, **2**.

Hartmann, H., Kris, E. & Loewenstein, R. M. (1949). Notes on the theory of aggression. *Psychoanal. Study Child*, **3-4**.

Heimann, P. (1942). A contribution to the problem of sublimation and its relation to processes of internalization. *Int. J. Psycho-Anal.*, **23**.

Hendrick, I. (1942). Instinct and the ego during infancy. *Psychoanal. Quart.*, **11**.

Hendrick, I. (1943). Work and the pleasure principle. *Psychoanal. Quart.*, **12**.

REFERENCES

Hendrick, I. (1951). Early development of the ego: identification in infancy. *Psychoanal. Quart.*, **20**.

Isaacs, S. (1948). The nature and function of phantasy. In *Developments in Psycho-Analysis*, edited by J. Riviere. London: Hogarth Press, 1952.

Jacobson, E. (1946). The effect of disappointment on ego and super-ego formation in normal and depressive development. *Psychoanal. Rev.*, **33**.

Jacobson, E. (1953). Contribution to the metapsychology of cyclothymic depression. In *Affective Disorders*, edited by P. Greenacre. New York: International Universities Press.

Jahoda, M. (1958). *Current Concepts of Positive Mental Health.* New York: Basic Books.

Jones, E. (1911). The pathology of morbid anxiety. *Papers on Psycho-Analysis.* London: Baillière, Tindall & Cox; 4th ed., 1938.

Jones, E. (1925). Introduction to symposium on the relation of psycho-analytic theory to psycho-analytic technique. *Int. J. Psycho-Anal.*, **6**.

Jones, E. (1926). The origin and structure of the super-ego. *Papers on Psycho-Analysis.* London: Baillière, Tindall & Cox; 4th ed., 1938.

Jones, E. (1929). Fear, guilt and hate. *Papers on Psycho-Analysis.* London: Baillière, Tindall & Cox; 5th ed., 1948.

Jones, E. (1930). Psycho-analysis and psychiatry. *Ibid.*

Jones, E. (1932). The concept of a normal mind. *Ibid.*

Jones, E. (1936). Psycho-analysis and the instincts. *Ibid.*

Jones, E. (1946). A valedictory address. *Int. J. Psycho-Anal.*, **27**.

Jones, E. (1947). The genesis of the super-ego. *Papers on Psycho-Analysis.* London: Baillière, Tindall & Cox; 5th ed., 1948.

Kanzer, M. (1952). The transference neurosis of the Rat Man. *Psychoanal. Quart.*, **21**.

Klein, M. (1927). Symposium on child analysis. *Contributions to Psycho-Analysis 1921-1945.* London: Hogarth Press, 1948.

Klein, M. (1932). *The Psycho-Analysis of Children.* London: Hogarth Press.

Klein, M. (1935). A contribution to the psychogenesis of manic-depressive states. *Contributions to Psycho-Analysis 1921-1945.* London: Hogarth Press, 1948.

Klein, M. (1940). Mourning and its relation to manic-depressive states. *Ibid.*

Klein, M. (1945). The oedipus complex in the light of early anxieties. *Ibid.*

Klein, M. (1946). Notes on some schizoid mechanisms. *Developments in Psycho-Analysis*. London: Hogarth Press, 1952.

Klein, M. (1948). *Contributions to Psycho-Analysis 1921-1945*. London: Hogarth Press.

Klein, M. (1950). On the criteria for the termination of an analysis. *Int. J. Psycho-Anal.*, **31**.

Klein, M. (1952). *Developments in Psycho-Analysis*. London: Hogarth Press.

Knapp, P. H., Levin, S., McCarter, R. H., Wermer, H. & Zetzel, E. (1960). Suitability for psychoanalysis: a review of one hundred supervised analytic cases. *Psychoanal. Quart.*, **29**.

Knight, R. P. (1953). Borderline states. In *Psychoanalytic Psychiatry and Psychology*, edited by R. P. Knight & C. R. Friedman. New York: International Universities Press, 1954.

Kris, E. (1950). On preconscious mental processes. *Psychoanalytic Explorations in Art.* New York: International Universities Press, 1952.

Lagache, D. (1951). Quelques aspects du transfert. *Rev. franç. Psychanal.*, **15**.

Lampl-de Groot, J. (1963). Symptom formation and character formation. *Int. J. Psycho-Anal.*, **44**.

Lewin, B. D. (1950). *The Psychoanalysis of Elation*. New York: Norton.

Lewin, B. D. (1954). Sleep, narcissistic neurosis, and the analytic situation. *Psychoanal. Quart.*, **23**.

Loewald, H. W. (1951). Ego and reality. *Int. J. Psycho-Anal.*, **32**.

Loewald, H. W. (1960). On the therapeutic action of psychoanalysis. *Int. J. Psycho-Anal.*, **41**.

Loewenstein, R. M. (1940). The vital or somatic instincts. *Int. J. Psycho-Anal.*, **21**.

Macalpine, I. (1950). The development of the transference. *Psychoanal. Quart.*, **19**.

Mahler, M. S. (1952). On child psychosis and schizophrenia: autistic and symbiotic infantile psychoses. *Psychoanal. Study Child*, **7**.

Mahler, M. S. (1963). Thoughts about development and individuation. *Psychoanal. Study Child*, **18**.

Mahler, M. S. (1969). *On Human Symbiosis and the Vicissitudes of Individuation*, vol. 1. New York: International Universities Press; London: Hogarth Press.

Mahler, M. S. & LaPerriere, K. (1965). Mother-child interaction during separation-individuation. *Psychoanal. Quart.*, **34**.

Margolin, S. G. (1953). Genetic and dynamic psychophysiological determinants of pathophysiological processes. In *The Psychosomatic Concept in Psychoanalysis*, edited by F. Deutsch. New York: International Universities Press.

Modell, A. H. (1963). Primitive object relationships and the predisposition to schizophrenia. *Int. J. Psycho-Anal.*, **44**.

Nacht, S. & Racamier, P. C. (1960). Symposium on depressive illness. II. Depressive states. *Int. J. Psycho-Anal.*, **41**.

Ogilvie, H. (1949). In praise of idleness. *Brit. med. J.*, **1**.

Pear, T. H. (1948). Perspectives in modern psychology. *Brit. J. Psychol.*, **38**.

Radó, S. (1928). The problem of melancholia. *Int. J. Psycho-Anal.*, **91**.

Rank, B. (1949). Aggression. *Psychoanal. Study Child*, **3–4**.

Rank, B. & MacNaughton, D. (1950). A clinical contribution to early ego development. *Psychoanal. Study Child*, **5**.

Rank, O. (1924). *The Trauma of Birth.* New York: Brunner, 1952.

Rapaport, D. (1960). *The Structure of Pyschoanalytic Theory.* New York: International Universities Press.

Rapaport, D. (1967). *Collected Papers*, edited by M. M. Gill. New York and London: Basic Books.

Rapaport, D. & Gill, M. M. (1959). The points of view and assumptions of metapsychology. *Int. J. Psycho-Anal.*, **40**.

Reich, A. (1958). A character formation representing the interaction of unusual conflict solutions into the ego structure. Abstracted in panel: The psychoanalytic concept of character (rep. by A. F. Valenstein). *J. Amer. psychoanal. Assoc.*, **6**.

Reik, T. (1941). Aggression from anxiety. *Int. J. Psycho-Anal.*, **22**.

Ritvo, S. & Solnit, A. J. (1958). Influences of early mother-child interaction on identification processes. *Psychoanal. Study Child*, **13**.

Rosenberg, E. (1946). *See* Zetzel, E. Rosenberg (1946).

Rosenfeld, H. (1952). Transference-phenomena and transference-analysis in an acute catatonic schizophrenic patient. *Int. J. Psycho-Anal.*, **33**.

Schur, M. (1953). The ego in anxiety. In *Drives, Affects, Behavior*, edited by R. M. Loewenstein. New York: International Universities Press.

Schur, M. (1955). Comments on the metapsychology of somatization. *Psychoanal. Study Child*, **10**.

Spitz, R. A. (1945). Hospitalism: an inquiry into the genesis of psychiatric conditions in early childhood. *Psychoanal. Study Child*, **1**.

Spitz, R. A. (1946). Anaclitic depression: an inquiry into the genesis of psychiatric conditions in early childhood. *Psychoanal. Study Child*, **2**.

Spitz, R. A. (1956). Countertransference: comments on its varying role in the analytic situation. *J. Amer. psychoanal. Assoc.*, **4**.

Sterba, R. (1934). The fate of the ego in analytic therapy. *Int. J. Psycho-Anal.*, **15**.

Stone, L. (1961). *The Psychoanalytic Situation.* New York: International Universities Press.

Strachey, J. (1934). The nature of the therapeutic action of psycho-analysis. *Int. J. Psycho-Anal.*, **15**.

Tartakoff, H. (1958). Introduction to panel: The psychoanalytic concept of character. *J. Amer. psychoanal. Assoc.*, **6**.

Tartakoff, H. (1966). The normal personality in our culture and the Nobel Prize complex. In *Psychoanalysis—A General Psychology: Essays in Honor of Heinz Hartmann*, edited by R. M. Loewenstein *et al.* New York: International Universities Press.

Trotter, W. (1916). *Instincts of the Herd in Peace and War.* London: Benn; 2nd ed., 1919.

Waelder, R. (1937). The problem of the genesis of psychical conflict in earliest infancy. *Int. J. Psycho-Anal.*, **18**.

Waelder, R. (1954). Contribution to panel: Defence mechanisms and psychoanalytic technique. *J. Amer. psychoanal. Assoc.*, **2**.

Winnicott, D. W. (1955). Metapsychological and clinical aspects of regression within the psycho-analytical set-up. *Collected Papers.* London: Tavistock Publications, 1958.

Wisdom, J. O. (1961). A methodological approach to the problem of hysteria. *Int. J. Psycho-Anal.*, **42**.

Zetzel, E. Rosenberg (1946). An unusual neurosis following head injury. *Int. J. Psycho-Anal.*, **27**.

Zetzel, E. Rosenberg (1953). Reality trauma and reality sense. *Int. J. Psycho-Anal.*, **35**. (Abstract.)

Zetzel, E. Rosenberg (1964). Symptom formation and character formation: a contribution to discussion. *Int. J. Psycho-Anal.*, **45**.

Zetzel, E. Rosenberg (1965). Dynamics of the metapsychology of the aging process. In *Geriatric Psychiatry*, edited by M. A. Berezin & S. H. Cath. New York: International Universities Press.

Zilboorg, G. (1933). Anxiety without affect. *Psychoanal. Quart.*, **2**.

BIBLIOGRAPHY OF WRITINGS BY ELIZABETH R. ZETZEL

1940 (With E. Guttman.) Chronic neurotics and the outbreak of war. *Lancet*, **239**.

1943 A clinical contribution to the psychopathology of the war neuroses. *Int. J. Psycho-Anal.*, **24**. (Read to British Psycho-Analytical Society, 3 March 1943. Reprinted: *Ybk Psychoanal.*, **1**.)

1946 An unusual neurosis following head injury. *Int. J. Psycho-Anal.*, **27**. (Read to British Psycho-Analytical Society, 1 May 1946.)

1949 Anxiety and the capacity to bear it. *Int. J. Psycho-Anal.*, **30**. (Read to British Psycho-Analytical Society, 4 May 1949. Reprinted: *Ybk Psychoanal.*, **6**.)

1949 The changing functions of a psychiatric outpatient department. *Quart. Bull. Brit. psychol. Soc.*, **1**, no. 5.

1951 Observations on dynamic changes after prefrontal lobotomy. *Archs Neurol. Psychiat.*, **66**; *J. nerv. ment. Dis.*, **116**. (Read to Boston Society of Psychiatry and Neurology, 17 May 1951.)

1952 Psychoanalytic observations regarding the dynamic effects of prefrontal lobotomy. *Bull. Amer. psychoanal. Assoc.*, **8**.

1953 The dynamic basis of supervision. *J. soc. Casework*, **34**.

1953 The depressive position. In *Affective Disorders*, edited by P. Greenacre. New York: International Universities Press.

1953 Contribution to discussion. In *The Psychosomatic Concept in Psychoanalysis*, edited by F. Deutsch. New York: International Universities Press.

1953 Panel report: The traditional psychoanalytic technique and its variations. *J. Amer. psychoanal. Assoc.*, **1**.

1954 Reality trauma and reality sense. (Abstract.) *Int. J. Psycho-Anal.*, **35**. (Read at 18th Congress of the International Psycho-Analytical Association, London, 1953.)

1954 Panel report: Defence mechanisms and psychoanalytic technique. *J. Amer. psychoanal. Assoc.*, **2**.

1955 The concept of anxiety in relation to the development of psychoanalysis. *J. Amer. psychoanal. Assoc.*, **3**.

1956 Current concepts of transference. *Int. J. Psycho-Anal.*, **37**. (Read at 19th Congress of the International Psycho-Analytical Association, Geneva, 1955.)

1956 An approach to the relation between concept and content in psychoanalytic theory: with special reference to the work of Melanie Klein and her followers. *Psychoanal. Study Child*, **11**.

1958 Therapeutic alliance in the psychoanalysis of hysteria. Abstracted in panel: Technical aspects of transference (rep. by D. Leach). *J. Amer. psychoanal. Assoc.*, **6**.

1958 Ernest Jones: his contribution to psycho-analytic theory. *Int. J. Psycho-Anal.*, **39**. (Adapted from papers read to British Psycho-Analytical Society, 19 March 1958, and American Psycho-analytical Association, 11 May 1958.)

1960 Criteria for analysability. (Panel of the American Psycho-analytic Association.) *J. Amer. psychoanal. Assoc.*, **8**.

1960 Introduction to symposium on depressive illness. *Int. J. Psycho-Anal.*, **41**. (Read at 21st Congress of the International Psycho-Analytical Association, Copenhagen, 1959.)

1960 The problem of accreditation. *Bull. Philadelphia Assoc. Psycho-anal.*, **10**.

1960 (With P. H. Knapp *et al.*) Suitability for psychoanalysis: a review of one hundred supervised analytic cases. *Psychoanal Quart.*, **29**.

1961 Melanie Klein 1882-1960. *Psychoanal. Quart.*, **30**.

1964 Symptom formation and character formation: a contribution to discussion. *Int. J. Psycho-Anal.*, **45**. (Read at 23rd Congress of the International Psycho-Analytical Association, Stockholm, 1963.)

1964 Closing address: First Pan-American Congress for Psycho-analysis. *Int. J. Psycho-Anal.*, **45**.

1964 Discussion of paper by Herbert Rosenfeld: 'Object relations of the acute schizophrenic patient in the transference situation'. In *Recent Research on Schizophrenia*, edited by P. Solomon & B. C. Glueck. Washington, D.C.: American Psychiatric Association.

1965 The use and misuse of psychoanalysis in psychiatric evaluation and psychotherapeutic practice. In *Proceedings of the 6th International Congress of Psychotherapy*, edited by M. Pines & T. Spoerri. Basel and New York: Karger.

1965 Depression and the incapacity to bear it. In *Drives, Affects, Behavior*, vol. 2, edited by M. Schur. New York: International Universities Press.

1965 Dynamics of the metapsychology of the aging process. In *Geriatric Psychiatry*, edited by M. A. Berezin & S. H. Cath. New York: International Universities Press.

1965 The effects of psychotherapy. *Int. J. Psychiat.*, **1**, nos. 1–2.

1965 The theory of therapy in relation to a development model of the psychic apparatus. *Int. J. Psycho-Anal.*, **46**. (Read at 22nd Congress of the International Psycho-Analytical Association, Edinburgh, 1961, and to the American Psychoanalytic Association, December 1963.)

1966 The analytic situation. In *Psychoanalysis in the Americas*, edited by Robert E. Litman. New York: International Universities Press. (Read at the First Pan-American Congress for Psychoanalysis, Buenos Aires, 1964.)

1966 The predisposition to depression. *Canad. psychiat. Assoc. J.*, **11** (suppl.). (Read at the McGill University Research Conference on The Depressive Group of Illnesses, February 1965.)

1966 Drugs or psychotherapy—William Sargant. In *Psychiatric Drugs*, edited by P. Solomon. New York: Grune & Stratton. (Read at Conference on Psychiatric Drugs, Boston State Hospital, 1965.)

1966 In memoriam: Max Gitelson 1902–1965. *J. Amer. psychoanal. Assoc.*, **14**.

1966 1965: Additional notes upon a case of obsessional neurosis: Freud 1909. *Int. J. Psycho-Anal.*, **47**. (Read at 24th Congress of the International Psycho-Analytical Association, Amsterdam, 1965.)

1966 Transference in psychotherapy. (Presented at Symposium on the Role of Transference in Psychotherapy, Department of Psychiatry, Tufts University School of Medicine, 20 May 1966.)

1967 (With J. Ewalt *et al.*) Long-term treatment of chronic schizophrenia. *Int. J. Psychiat.*, **4**.

1967 The relationship of defence to affect and its tolerance. In *The Unconscious Today*. (Volume of essays in honour of Max Schur; to appear.) (Read at the Annual Meeting of the American Psychoanalytical Association, 1967.)

1968 The so called good hysteric. *Int. J. Psycho-Anal.*, **49**. (Read at 25th Congress of the International Psycho-Analytical Association, Copenhagen, 1967.)

1968 Represión de la experiencia traumática y proceso de aprendizaje. (Repression of traumatic experience and the learning experience.) *Rev. Psicoanál.*, **25**. (Read at the Fall Meeting of the American Psychoanalytical Association, 1964. Abstracted in panel: Memory and repression, rep. by W. G. Niederland. *J. Amer. psychoanal. Assoc.*, **13** (1965).)

1968 Discussion of 'Psychoanalytic theory and the teaching of dynamic psychiatry' by R. M. Loewenstein. In *The Teaching of Dynamic Psychiatry*, edited by G. L. Bibring. New York: International Universities Press. (Contribution to the Beth Israel Hospital Symposium, 1964.)

1969 The analytic process. In *Psicoanálisis en las Américas*, edited by L. Grinberg *et al*. Buenos Aires: Paidós.

1969 96 Gloucester Place: some personal recollections. *Int. J. Psycho-Anal.*, **50**.

1970 Discussion of 'Towards a basic psychoanalytic model' by Joseph Sandler and W. G. Joffe. *Int. J. Psycho-Anal.*, **51**. (Presented at 26th Congress of the International Psycho-Analytical Association, Rome, 1969.)

BOOK REVIEWS

1932 *Mind and Money—A Psychologist Looks at the Crisis* by J. T. MacCurdy. *Int. J. Psycho-Anal.*, **13**.

1933 *Sin and the New Psychology* by C. E. Barbour. *Int. J. Psycho-Anal.*, **14**.

1934 *A New Physiological Psychology* by W. Burridge. *Int. J. Psycho-Anal.*, **15**.

1938 *Modern Psychology in Practice* by W. L. Neustatter. *Int. J. Psycho-Anal.*, **19**.

1938 *The Management of Early Infancy; Puberty and Adolescence; The Psychological Approach; The Neurotic Character;* by E. J. Partridge *et al. Int. J. Psycho-Anal.*, **19**.

1938 *Love and Happiness* (*Intimate Problems of the Modern Woman*) by I. M. Hotep. *Int. J. Psycho-Anal.*, **19**.

1941 *Clinical Studies in Psychopathology: A Contribution to the Aetiology of Neurotic Illness* by H. V. Dicks. *Int. J. Psycho-Anal.*, **22**.

1955 Recent British approaches to problems of early mental development. (*Developments in Psycho-Analysis* by Melanie Klein *et al.*; *Primary Love and Psycho-Analytic Technique* by M. Balint; *Psycho-Analytical Studies of the Personality* by R. D. Fairbairn; 'The so-called English school of psychoanalysis' by E. Bibring.) *J. Amer. psychoanal. Assoc.*, **3**.

1958 *Envy and Gratitude: A Study of Unconscious Sources* by Melanie Klein. *Psychoanal. Quart.*, **27**.

1963 The significance of the adaptive hypothesis for psychoanalytic theory and practice. (*Psychoanalysis of Behavior: Collected Papers* by S. Radó & G. E. Daniels.) *J. Amer. psychoanal. Assoc.*, **11**.

1965 *Introduction to the Work of Melanie Klein* by H. Segal. *Psychoanal. Quart.*, **34**.

1966 *Personality Structure and Human Interaction* by H. Guntrip. *Psychiatry*, **29**.

1967 Psychosis and the very young infant. (*Psychotic States* by H. A. Rosenfeld.) *Contemp. Psychol.*, **12**.

1967 *Psychoanalytic Supervision* by J. Fleming & T. F. Benedek. *J. nerv. ment. Dis.*, **145**.

1967 *Psychoanalysts in Training—Selection and Evaluation* by H. R. Klein. *Psychosom. Med.*, **29**.

1968 *The Psychoanalysis of Dreams* by A. Garma. *Psychoanal. Quart.*, **37**.

1969 *The Technique and Practice of Psychoanalysis*, vol. 1, by R. R. Greenson. *Int. J. Psycho-Anal.*, **50**.

INDEX

INDEX

INDEX